Marriage and Fertility in Chile

Dellplain Latin American Studies

Marriage and Fertility in Chile: Demographic Turning Points in the Petorca Valley, 1840–1976

Robert McCaa

Recent population increases in Latin America have forced population experts to search for historical precedents and to examine the latest demographic data in an attempt to forecast the likely course of future trends. This book is the first demographic study of a Latin American community based on the family genealogy method developed by French historians. Providing both a historical view and a consideration of very recent population developments, the author shows that despite strictures of the Catholic Church and popular attitudes favoring procreation, Chileans consistently have been quite sensitive to population pressures.

According to Dr. McCaa, a century ago the people of Petorca responded to worsening conditions by delaying marriage and by moving to more prosperous regions; now they are reacting to Latin America's modern demographic revolution by consciously curtailing reproduction. Dr. McCaa concludes that the slogan that emerged from the World Population Conference in Bucharest in 1979--"Modernization is the best contraceptive"--certainly is true in Chile, but finds it surprising how little modernization is necessary to bring about a substantial decline in fertility. Moreover, he points out that perceptions of the population explosion in Latin America are distorted to a degree by the fact that the fertility decline has been accompanied by an increase in the proportion of women who marry and a lowering of the average age at the time of marriage. These developments, he says, disguise the real decline in fertility and will continue to do so until it becomes quite noticeable.

Dr. Robert McCaa is assistant professor of history at the University of Minnesota. A population historian, he has studied demography and statistics in the United States and England.

Marriage and Fertility in Chile

Demographic Turning Points in the Petorca Valley, 1840–1976

Robert McCaa

Dellplain Latin American Studies, No. 14

Routledge
Taylor & Francis Group
LONDON AND NEW YORK

First published 1983 by Westview Press

Published 2018 by Routledge
52 Vanderbilt Avenue, New York, NY 10017
2 Park Square, Milton Park, Abingdon, Oxon OX14 4RN

Routledge is an imprint of the Taylor & Francis Group, an informa business

Library of Congress Cataloging in Publication Data
McCaa, Robert.
Marriage and fertility in Chile.
(Dellplain Latin American studies; no. 14)
Bibliography: p.
Includes index.
1. Fertility, Human--Chile--Petorca River Valley--History. 2. Marriage--Chile--Petorca River Valley--History. I. Title. II. Series.
HB976.P47M32 1983 304.6'32'098324 83-3494

ISBN 13: 978-0-367-01971-6 (hbk)

Contents

Tables

Figures

Acknowledgements

This study represents one of the first completed applications of family reconstitution methods to a non-European cultural area. I planned to study the population history of the community from 1720 forward, but the poor state of the earliest records and exhaustion of available resources forced the exclusion of both the colonial quantitative data and most nondemographic topics. The seven years that I have needed to complete the task are a reflection of the technical complexities of applying the method to Chilean registry books and my rather costly education through research.

Many people and organizations supported my work. My greatest debts are to my family--Wanda, Steven and Kennon--who sacrificed companionship, time and standard of living and endured my scholarly obsessions with extraordinary patience and understanding. Dr. Robert N. Burr, my thesis adviser, gave me freedom and professional support essential for the realization of a project of this type. John D. Durand stimulated my interest in population and provided much needed advice. Rolando Mellafe, Mario Góngora, René Salinas Mesa and the staff of the Instituto de Historia y Geografía of the Universidad Católica de Valparaíso taught me much about Chilean archives, parish registers, and Chilean history in general. My single greatest scholarly debt is to the staff of the Cambridge Group for the History of Population and Social Structure, in particular E. A. Wrigley, R. S. Schofield, and R. Davies, who salvaged the project when all seemed lost. Stuart Schwartz and my colleagues in the Department of History, University of Minnesota, provided the strongly supportive ambience necessary for completing the manuscript. Some of these people may be dismayed at certain errors and omissions which they sought to help me avoid but with limited success.

Angela Carreño, an accountant in Petorca, and Adriana Gonzalez, the statistician at the Petorca Hospital, helped greatly in the tedious collection of data and generally kept the project going while I was in Petorca. I am especially grateful for their hospitality, advice on local matters and friendship. Doña Marta Polanco, the Petorca Civil Registrar, the directors of the Central Civil Registry Office and Padre José Jaramillo graciously provided access to parish and civil register archives. Odette Tacla Chamy made available 1970 census data. The staff of the National Archives graciously provided every facility; I am particularly grateful for the opportunity to search the unorganized sections for nineteenth-century census manuscripts.

This project depended upon many sponsors: The Foreign Area Fellowship Program of the American Council of Learned Societies and the Social Sciences Research Council, the Fulbright-Hays program, and the Population Council (Grant numbers D70.0132C and D73.030C) provided generous support at various times. The Centro de Computación of the Universidad Católica (de Chile) and Empresa de Comunicaciones del Estado provided (and indirectly subsidized) excellent services. The Computer Laboratory of Cambridge University made available almost unlimited computer time and professional software support. The University Computer Center (Minnesota) awarded sufficient funds to generate most of the final tables. To these people and institutions I express my gratitude.

R. M.

Abbreviations

GP	Gobernación de Petorca Archivo de la Intendencia de Aconcagua, San Felipe
JP	Archivo Judicial de Petorca Archivo Nacional, Santiago
NP	Archivo Notarial de Petorca* Archivo Nacional
DP	Archivo del Departamento de Petorca Archivo Nacional
CPGEN	Capitanía General Archivo Nacional
FV	Fondo Varios Archivo Nacional
MH	Ministerio de Hacienda Archivo Nacional
MI	Ministerio del Interior Archivo Nacional
INE	Instituto Nacional de Estadística (earlier designations include Servicio Nacional de Censos y Estadística, Oficina Central de Estadística, etc.)

*All references to Notarial documents after 1880 (i.e. volumes numbered greater than 1879) are located in the Notary Office in Petorca.

1 Population Change in the Petorca Valley and Elsewhere

The modern rise of population in Latin America confounds demographic theorists and exasperates social planners. The source of the surging rates of population growth is evident to everyone: a singularly, unprecedented decline in mortality with no apparent adjustment in fertility. For more than two decades, following the destruction of the traditional population equilibrium, the prospects for dampening growth rates have appeared dim. Population experts have cast about for historical precedents and the latest demographic data to divine the likely course of future trends. According to some analysts the historical experiences of other cultures are too diverse at best or, even worse, irrelevant to provide clues to the evolution of Latin American populations. At the same time contradictory conclusions are deduced from the same data by competent specialists.

This case study of population change in the Petorca Valley delineates the process of transition from a traditional demographic regime to a modern one. It is a study of the diffusion of population behavior and attitudes from modern, urban social groups to country-folk. The story began in Chile at least a century ago and has climaxed only in the present decade. The process remains unfinished.

None of the controversies over the nature of the demographic transition or the validity of the theory will be resolved by the analysis of a single community. The bindings of time and space are too tight for generalizations derived from an insignificant population to withstand the excessive strains imposed by grand theories. Nevertheless the study of relationships between demographic and social variables and the relative frequency of population differentials in a single community may assist our understanding the larger process of demographic modernization.

Given popular images of traditional populations, the diversity of marriage, family, and childbearing patterns found in the Petorca Valley over a century ago must be surprising. When the population history of Chile is written, if the demographic behavior of Petorcans provides any insights, it will likely show that the dissimilarities in demographic behavior rooted in the distant past have gradually radiated from city to village and, lately, to farm and mine. A pattern of behavior diffusing from social elites to the masses best describes the population changes experienced by Petorcans over the past century.

THE DEMOGRAPHIC TRANSITION

The story fits snugly into the classic demographic transition theory. The original theory's vagueness about the timing, pace, and interrelatedness of demographic changes--a liability in terms of its predictive power--becomes an asset for analyzing the past. In the first statement of the theory almost a half century ago, Warren S. Thompson sought to succinctly describe the demographic stages through which the Western European cultural area had passed--a process which he believed began in the early nineteenth century and only reached a climax after the First World War.[1] Thompson portrayed the story in three sequential, evolutionary phases. In the first stage a demographic equilibrium producing modest growth had been maintained through high fertility counterbalanced by high, if variable, mortality. In the second stage the rate of population increase temporarily spurted upward as mortality levels declined precipitously with little immediate adjustment in natality behavior. Finally a new homeostasis was achieved; the population balance sheet showed once again moderate rates of natural increase as fertility fell to historic lows.

Through a slow process of intellectual accretions, Thompson's generalizations have become a full-blown theory of "development or modernization." Thought on the demographic transition theory, because of its widespread currency and rather shallow foundations in empirical research, is diverse indeed. Some argue that it is neither good theory--it fails to delineate systematically the relationships between population change and broader social and economic developments--nor an accurate description of an historical process--the European experiences described by the recent generation of historical demographers are much too diverse to fit within a crude, mechanistic paradigm.[2] Nevertheless, according to a recent report by the Secretary General of the United Nations, ". . . the fact remains that every population that has experienced the impact of modernization has much lower fertility and mortality than before it was subject to such economic and social development."[3]

One of the principal objections is that there is no specification of linkages between social and economic modernization and fertility change. There seem to be no consistent levels of urbanization, education, industrialization, or even mortality which inevitably insure fertility decline. Moreover European population history indicates that a nonquantifiable cultural dimension conditions the association between social and economic variables and demographic change.[4]

Dudley Kirk and Frank Oeschli recently attempted to surmount these objections and reassess the validity of the theory.[5] They argue that much research on testing the theory has been marred by incorrect model specification and poor statistical procedures. Given the conditioning effects of culture, they propose to analyze demographic change within a single cultural area, Latin America, instead of across many regions which has often been the strategy. With regard to statistical procedures, instead of multiple regression or factor analysis, they propose an elegant, theoretically inspired transformation of social, demographic, and economic indicators into a development index. Finally, instead of blindly regressing all quantifiable variables against demographic rates, Kirk and Oeschli elaborate the theory, specify substantive relations, and carefully operationalize the research hypotheses on the basis of the theoretical model. They conclude that currently available evidence for a set of over twenty Latin American countries strongly supports the theory. Invariably countries with the highest levels of development have the lowest levels of mortality and fertility.

Under Kirk's direction, Stephen Beaver has completed the most detailed analysis and amplification of the theory in Latin America.[6] He finds support for the demographic transition concept and for many hypotheses derived therefrom. Probably the most significant finding to emerge is that rates of natality decline have become extremely rapid wherever the fertility decline has begun. Changes in birth rates are decidedly related to economic development, although the relationship with the crude death rate is not.[7]

Why should fertility behavior change with development? Richard Easterlin, incorporating the contributions of classical economics and sociology, has authored an elegant paradigm to explain fertility change at the family and individual level.[8] The determining factors, the linkages between modernization at the macro-level and fertility behavior of individuals, are the demand for children and the production of children. In a traditional demographic regime, the desire for children typically exceeds what most couples are able to produce. Subfecundity, illness, cultural taboos, absences of spouses, infant and adult mortality, and the like suppress the ability of most parents to meet their perceived economic and social need for children. At that stage, fertility performance is largely the product of social and biological forces--rarely the conscious choice of individuals. Modernization acts to inhibit the demand for children at the same time that parents' ability to produce offspring, particularly live descendants, improves greatly. At the point where the production of children exceeds demand, motivation for fertility control is generated.

Although Easterlin sketches the relationship between the process of modernization--urbanization, mass education, income growth, the production of new goods, etc.--and its effect on the production and consumption of children, the principal criticism of the appropriateness of the model for third world countries is directed precisely at the mode of contemporary modernization. For many years the fashion among demographers and other social scientists has been to lambast the theory as culture and time bound. The contemporary pattern of modernization differs markedly from that of nineteenth-century Europe, according to the critics.[9] Eduardo Arriaga has developed one of the most cogent, extensively researched critiques for Latin America.[10] He argues that contrary to European experiences mortality changes in Latin America often have taken place in spite of the lagging pace of social and economic development. The recent transition has been achieved cheaply, by the precipitous importation of modern medical and sanitation technologies without the social and economic infrastructures necessary to effect a decline in fertility. The European mortality transition was "earned"; economic, social, and demographic conditions were modernized in unison. An educated, prosperous work force and state bureaucracy were essential for realizing advances in survivorship and, at the same time, ensuring a predisposition toward a reduction in fertility. The process was an incremental one, occurring over decades, even generations.

In contrast, mortality changes in Latin America have been extremely abrupt, unprecedented for their velocity and scale. Arriaga demonstrates that, for Chile in particular and Latin America generally in recent decades, the changes were so rapid that people's life chances, like fine Chilean wines, improved as they aged. However, the advances were not accompanied by substantial social or economic changes, according to Arriaga. They were "unearned." Therefore it would be unwise to expect Latin American fertility trends to repeat any Western European pattern.[11]

In fact, Latin American fertility trends have not replicated European experiences. As Beaver noted, where natality declines have occurred they have been unprecedented in terms of both scale and velocity,[12] just as Arriaga demonstrated for mortality changes.

FERTILITY TRANSITION IN CHILE

The evolution of Chilean fertility patterns since the 1929 Depression are very clear today, now that a great and--according to the transition theory--irreversible decline in natality has occurred. Nevertheless, a few years ago demographers were hard pressed to anticipate accurately the likely course of Chilean fertility. Without a theory of population dynamics, demographers were reduced to making mechanical population projections. One of the most extensive, thorough reviews of Chilean demographic data in the early 1960s completely missed the mark in estimating fertility levels for the subsequent decade. Even the most liberal hypothesis, one considered very unlikely by the estimator, was about 33 percent too high. The hypothesized crude birth rate for 1970 was thirty-two; the actual rate at that date was twenty-four, a decline of 30 percent in less than a decade.[13]

Initial increases in birth rates, accurately predicted by Arriaga for the intermediate stage of mortality decline, were quickly reversed, contrary to the expectations of those who doubted the relevance of the demographic transition for Latin America. Within a single decade fertility rates plummetted to unprecedented lows; today Chilean birth rates are closer to those of the United States than to Chilean rates in the not too distant past.[14]

Declines in Petorcan fertility rates have lagged much behind national changes, just as the mortality declines were delayed in the valley. As one of the most impoverished communities in the region, one should expect that demographic change would reach the valley relatively late.

If Chilean fertility trends are clear, the demographic interrelations producing them are obscure and have not been thoroughly analyzed. The principal demographic explanations for rising rates in the 1950s has been, on the one hand, the increased survival of spouses and, on the other, age structural shifts favoring the fecund age groups of the population.[15] The demographic correlates of the natality change are much more complex. One of the most significant elements in this story is the extraordinarily flexible fertility behavior of Chilean women. On the one hand, interpretations of fertility change which stress changing age composition or prolongation of marital unions imply that natality increases are a statistical artifact which would disappear with the use of age-specific marital fertility rates and not the result of any genuine increase in the conception rate. On the other hand, fertility increases are perceived as real both for the individual and the population as an aggregate; increased conceptions are interpreted as simply the realization of fertility potential which, in an earlier epoch, were prematurely terminated by the disruptive effect of adult mortality.

The Petorca data indicates a substantial rise in marital fertility in the first years of the mortality transition. Moreover, a reworking of the national data indicates that natality within marriage increased perhaps 10 percent or more for the entire country during the first decade following the greatest improvements in survivalhood (1940-1949). Finally, the upward surge in marital fertility rates occurred precisely when the nuptiality transition--of younger ages at marriage and greater proportions ever-marrying--reached its greatest intensity. The direct effects of mortality, biological fecundity, and nuptiality pushed the Chilean rate of natural increase to the highest levels ever. Nevertheless, within a decade it was over.

The great natality decline which occurred in the 1960s was also the result of changes in conception rates. This was no statistical artifact. Nuptial rates did not decline; Chileans did not delay marriage; nor did celibacy increase. Quite the contrary, the nuptial propensities of the 1950s were extended and intensified in the following decade. Marriage rates did not peak until 1971. The natality decline occurred almost wholly through the conscious control of conception within marriage.

Why have these developments remained obscure? The analysis of population change in Latin America, particularly with regard to testing the validity of the demographic transition theory, has too long been clouded by the use of confusing crude measures. The technical sophistication of much demographic analysis notwithstanding, aggregative, cross-national research on the modernization of fertility in Latin America continues to be fought with the weakest tools available, specifically crude birth rates and general child-woman ratios.[16] Given the important disturbances caused by the transition to lower mortality--the proportion of the population in the youngest and oldest age groups increases relatively faster than for those in the fecund ages--crude rates must seem singularly inappropriate. If the effects of modernization on Chilean family formation patterns are replicated in other Latin American populations, demographic indicators which control for both age and marital structure are essential for accurately divining demographic modernization.[17]

In the case of Mexico, for example, which has aroused much interest because of its soaring rates of natural increase and was the recent subject of yet another "proof" of the failure of the demographic transition to indicate the path of fertility change in a non-European cultural area,[18] the evolution of crude rates, if analyzed at all, should be interpreted imaginatively rather than mechanically. If the demographic transition theory is correct, the consequences and correlates of modernization for the Latin American cultural area should be an increase in the frequency of stable family unions, a prolongation of marriages and a rise in the natural procreative potential of couples. As a result of improvements in public health and increasing maternal morbidity, fertility should surge upward until people begin to control conception risks through abstinence, <u>coitus interruptus</u> or more technical means of contraception. One should expect the immediate effects of fertility within marriage to force high crude birth rates even higher. In the presence of a mortality transition, static natality rates following a sustained mortality decline would seem to indicate controlled fertility, at least to the extent of counterbalancing the increases expected from rising nuptiality, improved maternal morbidity and fecundity, and the prolongation of marital unions.

VARIETIES OF POPULATION CHANGE IN THE PAST

The story of fertility change in the Petorca Valley is intriguing, demonstrating the finely tuned interaction between the four principal components of population: marriage, fertility, mortality, and migration. Nineteenth-century fertility rates of Petorcan women were high when compared with most natural fertility populations, but not the highest. At the middle of the last century Petorca women marrying at age twenty and completing the entire fertility cycle bore 8.5 children on the average, a figure slightly greater than that for the Norman parish Crulai (8.2 for women marrying during 1674-1742) but considerably less than that for French Canadian women in the early eighteenth century (10.8).[19] Of course, this is an ordinary, expected finding for rural Chile. However, it is somewhat surprising to encounter fertility differentials at that date. Moreover, after adjustments for underenumeration, with each successive marriage cohort a pattern emerges of a steady, slow rise in fertility lasting over a century. The greatest increase in fertility is found for women marrying within fifteen years after the onset of the Great Depression. After 1945 a substantial decline in marital fertility occurred, several years before the initiation of a birth control program at the local hospital.

The rates of natality change for select subgroups of the population show significant differences. Declines are greatest for the occupational and educational elite and smallest for poorer women from farm families. In fact, total fertility rates for married women with bastard origins increased to the highest levels recorded for any group in the history of the valley (10.0 total marital fertility ages 20-49 compared with 7.4 for women whose husbands worked in white-collar jobs). The extraordinary impoverishment and comparatively low standard of living of the valley's inhabitants notwithstanding, a fertility transition began very soon after substantial advances in mortality control.

In spite of the apparent social homogeneity of the residents of the valley given its overwhelmingly rural character, occupation and educational differentials are impressively correlated with the childbearing experiences of Petorcan women. In fact, fertility differentials are noticeable from the earliest period studied. Literate Petorcans have had measurably lower fertility than their illiterate neighbors for more than a century. Similarly, on average, spouses from legitimate families have always borne slightly fewer children than those with illegitimate origins. However, the greatest differentials in fertility are found between occupational groups. For more than a century husbands with civil occupations generally sired fewer children than those working in agriculture and mining. The highly suspicious reliability of the data notwithstanding, these patterns are so systematic that they must be genuine.

Does this mean that some social groups consciously restricted their fertility to a measurable degree in the distant past? Or are the differentials the result of some particular social controls or perhaps biological differences dependent on social class? The answer for the most recent generation is clear and unequivocal: a substantial portion of the petite bourgeoisie consciously controlled their fertility in the 1950s and 1960s. Plots of the age-specific fertility rates for this group display the concave pattern typical of populations practicing contraception. Before 1945 conscious fertility control was exercised too infrequently or ineffectively to be determined conclusively. The shape of the fertility curves for the occupational elite dating from the 1860s may indicate some partial control, which over the years becomes more pronounced; however, the largest changes clearly occur after 1945. In fact, the total fertility rates for women marrying in the 1930s were closer to those of their grandmothers than to those of their own daughters. Fertility rates for most of the cohorts formed in the interim 1863-1945 are intermediate between those for 1860 and 1945; nevertheless, the 1930 cohort shows a return to the higher fertility pattern of a century earlier.

If conscious fertility controls are discarded as unlikely for past generations how may one account for observed fertility differences? They are not likely the result of error. Registration should be best for the groups with precisely the lowest fertility rates. If hypothetical adjustments were made, in addition to the corrections directly derived from empirical information, they would have to be greater for the illiterate population than the literate, thereby increasing the disparities between the two groups. Educated villagers perhaps experienced poorer health conditions because of crowding, the more prolific spread of infectious and contagious diseases, contaminated water supplies, and the like. Similarly they may have had lowered rates of coital intercourse because of the intermittent absence of husbands attending to business concerns outside the valley or other social reasons. Perhaps the reduced conception rates had a genetical basis. Consanguineous marriages were extremely common in the valley, particularly amongst the elite, as a means of preventing the fragmentation of the family inheritance. The biological endogamy rates for Petorca (based on 2926 marriages, 1840-1894) are higher than any reported by Sutter for nineteenth-century French parishes registering more than 100 marriages. The ratio for Petorca during this period was 246 ("Wright's F") compared with a range of 3 to 231 for twenty-seven French parishes.[20] If the causes of the fertility rate differences are impossible to decipher, their existence should not necessarily be questioned. Charbonneau also found noticeable natural fertility differences between occupations for Tourouvre dating from 1665.[21]

The Petorca fertility and nuptiality data demonstrate that the categorization of demographic regimes as traditional and modern is a simplification. For well over a century Petorcans from socially distinct groups of families have exhibited heterogeneous fertility rates. Nevertheless, a dualistic categorization of the demographic history of the valley is substantively defensible because until recently all groups were characterized by a single pattern of natural fertility. Differences in both level and pattern of childbearing were between a very small elite (only fourteen families in the period 1840-1862) and the broad mass.

The process of differentiation did not accelerate until this century. At that time the basic demographic features of the community began to change greatly through gradual increments, reflecting the complex interplay of economic and social modernization and simultaneously stimulating a cumulative, sustained decline in mortality, an increase in marriage propensities, and a short-lived upsurge in fertility. Natality decline after 1970 was abrupt and precipitous. It began early in this century within the most advantaged households and by 1950 was measurable in the life histories of a large group of families. Hospital records for the 1960s show many women resorting to crudely induced abortions to prevent unwanted births. When the family planning program finally began in the valley in 1972 approximately 15 to 20 percent of obstetric and gynecologic admissions involved surgical interventions to extract fetal remains threatening the life of the mother. After 1972, for every one hundred births occurring in the hospital, there were seventy-five intrauterine contraceptive devices inserted and another fifty women provided with other kinds of modern contraceptives. From 1973 to 1976, 95 percent of pregnant women entering the local hospital were inscribed in an integrated family planning program.

Now demographic change has out-paced socioeconomic developments. Petorcans are rapidly acquiring modern demographic behavior while social and economic advances have virtually halted. The present generation of Petorcans have experienced within the time frame of two or three decades a revolutionary transformation in the fundamental biological processes of both death and birth. Their responses to a changing biological ambience have been conditioned by economic and social innovations inherent in the modernization process and have been ongoing, if somewhat sluggishly, for several generations. For Petorcans the demographic transition involved not only a mortality transition but both a fertility transition and a marriage transition.

The history of population change in the Petorca Valley shows that the modernization of populations is a wholistic, integral process, interactive and interdependent. At the same time that Petorcans began dying at much more advanced ages, they also began to marry much younger. Moreover, the incidence of permanent celibacy declined sharply. The implications of the marriage transition for population growth, which were true for the entire nation as well, were substantial. A greater proportion of women in the most fecund ages were in stable marital unions than probably at any other period in the valley's history. Secular marriage trends in the valley did not replicate those of nineteenth-century European populations; quite the contrary, their pattern more closely approximated nuptial patterns in the United States and Western Europe since 1945. The trend has been toward increasingly precocious, more universal stable marriage.

That great declines in fertility could be achieved by Chilean women in the face of declining celibacy and earlier marriage suggests the deliberativeness, the conscious choice favoring major fertility reductions. If during the 1950s fertility actually increased as a consequence of changes in the marital structure of the population and rising fertility rates within marriage, within a decade the increases evaporated and crude rates fell dramatically.

The demographic transition in the Petorca Valley has been realized only through substantial social and economic development. Without an educated populace, without an effective public bureaucracy, without rising standards of living, without improved social status of women, and without the spread of new styles of life, the pace of mortality change would have been slowed, its scale, meager. Likewise the spread of nuptiality to most of the adult population would have been economically unrealistic, fertility change, unnecessary.

For Petorcans the demographic transition was grounded in the educational reforms of more than a century ago, when President Manuel Montt, one of the valley's most accomplished native-sons, established and extended national public schools. Educational advances came slowly in the face of stark economic and fiscal realities. Truly universal schooling for most Petorca children has been achieved only recently.

For Petorcans the demographic transition was also rooted in institutionalized public health measures initiated through their own efforts over a century ago. The establishment of a smallpox sanitorium in 1801 and subsequent municipal policies encouraging widespread vaccination mark the first feeble efforts. For much of the nineteenth century local advances in public health were trivial, notwithstanding repeated efforts by the local citizenry to found a hospital, procure and retain a doctor, develop a wholesome, potable water supply, and generally improve the sanitary conditions of the community. When modern medicines became available in the valley, health workers operated from a hospital founded in the nineteenth century, cooperated with municipal governments which had struggled with health obstacles (both physical and fiscal) for generations, and consulted with parents and children educated in local schools established by the earliest residents and maintained by the national government.

A communication network, inexorably developed according to the economic needs of the community, allowed midwives, nurses, and doctors to provide medical services to the countryside. All weather cart roads, constructed in the mid-nineteenth century were gradually improved; the first asphalt pavement was laid in 1970. Until that time, the maternity service of the hospital was restricted to the village population. Afterwards, with the acquisition of ambulances, a greater proportion of parturitions occurred in the local hospital. Technological innovations and infrastructural developments were important conditioners of the pace and scale of the demographic transition. Without all weather roads and numerous salaried nurses and doctors, reductions in infant and child mortality were relatively modest. Later, with a change in government policy, the same facilities used to improve the public's health were also harnessed to encourage a decline in fertility.

To the extent that one can generalize from the population history of the Petorca Valley, both the advocates and the critics of the demographic transition are correct. The process of economic and social modernization in the valley has been anemic, partial, and perhaps abortive. Much of the cost of the mortality transition was borne elsewhere and many of the resultant social benefits accrued elsewhere as well. Nevertheless, even the reduced levels of modernization were sufficient to induce a major decline in fertility. Today Petorcans enjoy a modern demographic regime with only modest social and economic development.

NOTES

1. Warren S. Thompson, "Population," American Journal of Sociology, Vol. 34 (1929), pp. 959-975. See also C. P. Blacker, "Stages in Population Growth," Eugenics Review, Vol. 39 (1947), pp. 88-102; and, F. W. Notestein, "The Economics of Population and Food Supplies," Proceedings of the Eighth International Conference of Agricultural Economists (London, 1953), pp. 15-31.

2. Calvin Goldscheider, Population, Modernization and Social Structure (Boston, 1971), p. 14. Ansley J. Coale, "The Decline of Fertility in Europe from the French Revolution to World War II," in S. J. Behrman, Leslie Corsa, and Ronald Freedman (eds.), Fertility

and Family Planning: A World View (Ann Arbor, 1969), pp. 478-489. Massimo Livi-Bacci, "Fertility and Population Growth in Spain in the Eighteenth and Nineteenth Centuries," Daedalus, Vol. 97 (1968), pp. 523-535.

3. Secretary General of the United Nations, "Population Change and Economic and Social Development," in United Nations, The Population Debate: Dimensions and Perspectives. Papers of the World Population Conference Bucharest 1974 (New York, 1975), Vol. 1, p. 52.

4. Ansley J. Coale, "The Demographic Transition," in United Nations, The Population Debate, Vol. 1, pp. 347-355. Dudley Kirk and Frank Oeschli, "Modernization and the Demographic Transition in Latin America and the Caribbean," Economic Development and Cultural Change, Vol. 23 (1975), pp. 391-417. Michael S. Teitelbaum, "Importancia de la teoria de la transición demográfica para países en desarrollo," Demografía y Economía, Vol. 10 (1976), pp. 54-67.

5. Kirk and Oeschli, "Modernization and the," pp. 391-417.

6. Steven E. Beaver, Demographic Transition Theory Reinterpreted: An Application to Recent Natality Trends in Latin America (Lexington, MA, 1975), pp. 4-10.

7. Beaver, Demographic Transition Theory, p. 81, ff.

8. Richard A. Easterlin, "The Effects of Modernization on Family Reproductive Behavior," in United Nations, The Population Debate, Vol. 2, pp. 263-277.

9. Goldschneider, Population, Modernization and. See also, Etienne van de Walle, "Les enseignements de la transition demographique Européene," Cultures et Developpement, Vol. 7 (1975), pp. 575-585.

10. Eduardo E. Arriaga, "The Nature and Effects of Latin America's Non-Western Trend in Fertility," Demography, Vol. 7 (1970), pp. 483-501. See also his Mortality Decline and Its Demographic Effects in Latin America (Berkeley, 1970); and Eduardo E. Arriaga and Kingsley Davis, "The Pattern of Mortality Change in Latin America," Demography, Vol. 6 (1969), pp. 223-242.

11. Arriaga, "The Nature and," pp. 493-497.

12. Beaver, Demographic Transition Theory, p. 95, ff.

13. Johannes L. Sadie, "Población y mano de obra de Chile, 1930-1975," in Chile (Santiago, 1969), pp. 18-20. Servicio Nacional de Salud, Nacimientos, Anuario 1975 (Santiago, 1976), p. 2.

14. United Nations, Demographic Yearbook 1975 (New York, 1975), pp. 494-495.

15. Arriaga, Mortality Decline and, pp. 146-158.

16. Daniel A. Seiver, "Recent Fertility in Mexico: Measurement and Interpretation," Population Studies, Vol. 29 (1975), pp. 341-354. W. Whitney Hicks, "Economic Development and Fertility Change in Mexico, 1950-1970," Demography, Vol. 11 (1974), pp. 407-421.

17. Mayone J. Stycos (Human Fertility in Latin America: Sociological Perspectives [Ithaca, New York, 1968], pp. 202-215) noted the importance of studying fertility according to mating practices almost a decade ago. Only in the Caribbean area have demographers continued to take this challenge seriously. See G. W. Roberts, Fertility and Mating in Four West Indian Populations (Jamaica, 1975).

18. Seiver, "Recent Fertility in."

19. Roland Pressat, Demographic Analysis: Methods, Results and Applications (Chicago, 1972), p. 185.

20. J. Sutter and L. Tabah, "L'évolution des isolats de deux departments francais: Loit-et-Cher et Finistère," Population, Vol. 10 (1955), pp. 645-674.

21. Hubert Charbonneau, Tourouvre-au-Perche aux XVIIe et XVIIIe siecles: Etude de demographie historique (Paris, 1970), pp. 107-112.

2
Petorca, Pueblo of the Past

> Petorca was once the site of great riches because of its mining industry . . . but today there only remain traditions, which tell us of the boom of colonial times and even afterwards.
>
> Voz de Petorca, August 4, 1895

For more than a century Petorcans have longed for a return, if not to greatness, to at least the prosperity of times past. The mines, once rich in gold and copper, no longer provide the means to sustain the economy of the valley. With advances in mining technology in the late nineteenth century most small Chilean mining towns quickly decayed. The Chilean mining industry was painfully redirected toward the largest deposits where massive capital investments promised more generous profits to investors. Petorcans also dreamed of attracting foreign capital, rebuilding the mines with modern technology, and installing efficient smelters. German, French, and British experts visited the valley and inspected its ores. Some promised to rehabilitate El Bronze, Llahuín, Valdivia, or another of the old mines famous for the fortunes made for an earlier generation. Claims were staked, some money invested; but the mining boom never returned.[1]

AN ARID DEFILE

> The fact of having founded a settlement in a defile with no expanse whatsoever for making a living from agriculture, gives us motives for believing that . . . the settlement must have been impelled by some collosal riches.
>
> Voz de Petorca, August 4, 1895

The narrow canyon etched by the Petorca River's plunge to the sea has left little space for settlement. Three great ranch-farms have been staked out astride the largest alluvial fans, while small farmers struggle to habilitate strips of soil from niches scattered along the steep mountainside or perched precariously on the edge of the riverbed. Fields, still densely littered with stones after more than two centuries of tillage, are productive only in years of abundant moisture. By the workings of geological fate, the peaks which claustrophobically envelope the valley do not reach the heights of permanent snows (4,000 meters); consequently, by late spring the snows completely disappear and by midsummer the Petorca River virtually dries up. Many small irrigation canals, dikes, and dams, constructed to conserve and direct the available water, are useless during the frequent years of drought and light snows. Rivers to the north and the south of the Petorca have their origins on peaks thrusting above 4,500 meters and therefore enjoy a more abundant, constant flow of water in the driest years (Figure 2.1).[2]

Even in years of abundant rainfall, by midsummer the Petorca hillsides suggest a bleak moonscape. Barren slopes rising steeply from the river's edge provide little grazing for livestock. Goats are hard put to fatten on the spiny plants which cling in sparse clumps to the mountainside. The scant soils fail to conceal ever present porphyritic rock, which hint at vast mineral wealth hidden beneath but provide little sustenance for anything other than xerophytes. The subsoil consists almost entirely of Andean diorite.[3]

The extraordinarily dry climate and poor soils provide sufficient nutriment only for thorns and cactuses, although wherever the river widens some forests formed. Most forests, however, were cut over a century ago to fuel smelters or to make charcoal. Darwin noted thousands of Chilean palms near Las Palmas on the northwest corner of Petorca parish during his travels in Chile.[4]

Because of this hostile ambience, the valley was sparsely settled by the Spanish until the early eighteenth century. Communication with the outside was arduous. The tortuous path of the river made the natural exit unnecessarily long; moreover, there was no appropriate spot for a port near its mouth. Since the most frequented routes went over at least one mountain pass, the paths were too steep for oxcarts. Most cargo was moved by mule train. The transportation obstacles were only resolved in the first decade of this century with the construction of a long narrow tunnel across the Cuesta de la Grupa. This cut, which took over twenty years to complete, allowed easy access by railroad to La Ligua and then to the major port of Valparaiso, 150 kilometers to the southwest, or Santiago, 200 kilometers due south.[5]

SELECTING THE STUDY SITE

If geographical characteristics made settlement and economic growth difficult, they provide very good methodological reasons for selecting Petorca as the study site.

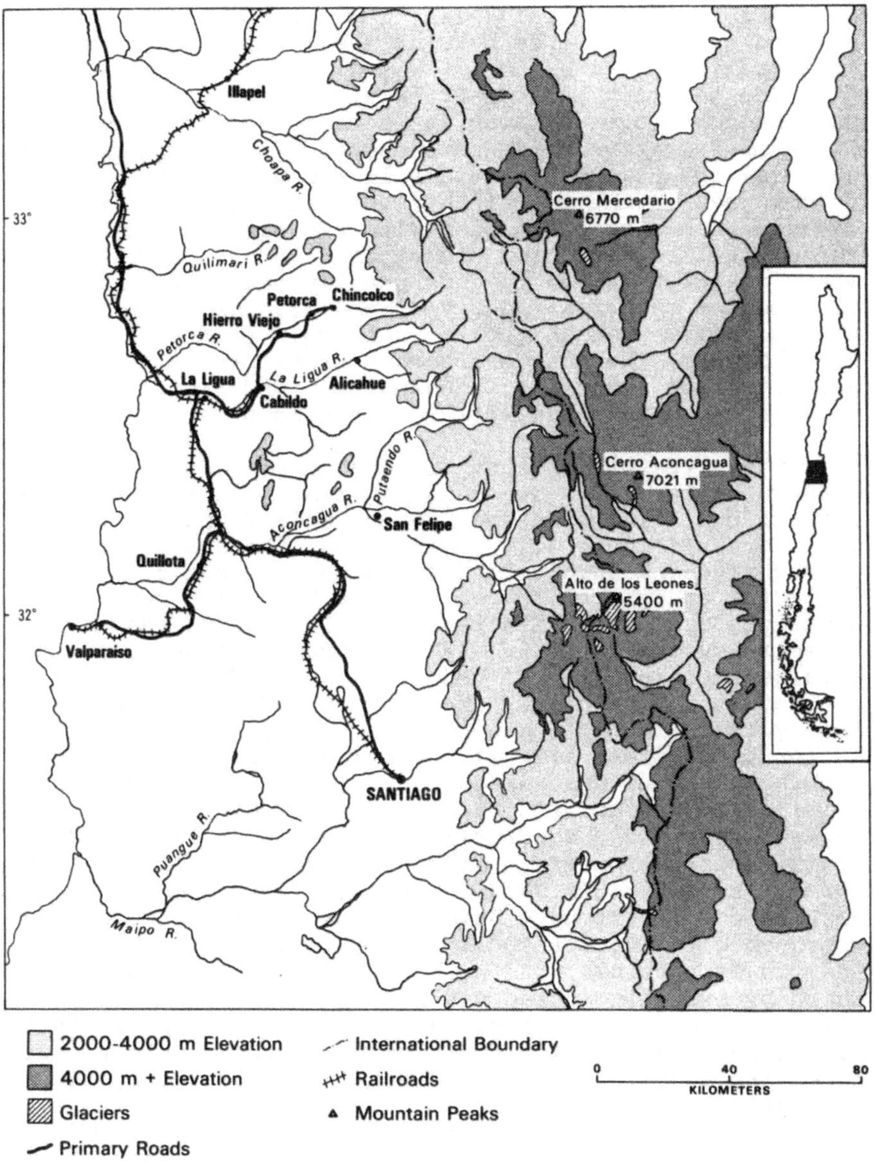

Figure 2.1 The Petorca Valley in a regional context

The valley's natural geographical boundaries ensured the concentration of settlement and constant administrative limits from the first attempted founding in 1753. Most Chilean communities are more spaciously situated and the activist state bureaucracy reformed administrative boundaries on many occasions. Moreover the geography of most parishes in the Central Valley invites population dispersal and an incongruence between their geographical and administrative confines.

The geographical constraints of the Petorca Valley have been too overwhelming for administrators to defy. Its administrative units have changed from partidos in the colonial era to subdelegations in the nineteenth century to communes in the twentieth. The vital events district evolved from a single parish with two secondary chapels to three civil registration districts. Both Petorca department, of which the valley has usually been the administrative center, and Aconcagua Province have been expanded and contracted, merged and split, submerged and redefined; nevertheless, the smallest census districts in the valley have retained remarkably unchanging boundaries from the earliest modern census (1813) to the most recent (1970) (Table 2.1).[6]

The situs of the study is the upper reaches of the Petorca Valley, from Quebrada de Yerba Loca in the extreme east to Puntilla Marín and Cuesta de la Grupa in the southwest corner (Figure 2.2). Because of the sheer magnitude of the research involved, a decision was made to further limit the study area to Petorca and Chincolco registration districts beginning with the establishment of the civil registry system in 1885. (The geographical unity of this area, stretching from El Peñon to the headwaters, was recognized in the original demarcations made by the Royal Surveyors in 1780.)[7] Nevertheless, baptisms were extracted for the western area of the parish through 1899. Although this area was reintegrated into the Petorca district in 1927, families' histories from Hierro Viejo, Pedegua, Artificio, and Frutillar were not analyzed for the civil registration era. With hindsight, all of the events for all subdistricts should have been extracted to avoid ensuing complications. Nevertheless, at the time it seemed reasonable to attempt to limit the reconstitution effort as much as possible; the work was reduced by about one-third by excluding these districts. People from Alicahue, a large fundo in the Ligua Valley, sometimes appear in the parish and registration books of the Petorca Valley, but they were also left aside because they appear only intermittently.

The size of Petorca parish is immense--over 1500 square kilometers--but the population is much more concentrated than these figures suggest.[8] The largest settlement is at Chincolco, where the population spreads over an area three kilometers wide by six long (Figure 2.3). Petorca Village, squeezed between river and mountain, has

TABLE 2.1
Administrative geography of the Petorca Valley

Administrative Unit				
Department		Petorca		
Parish		Petorca		
Subdelegation No.	2	3	4 (excluded after 1885-99)	5
Population - 1854	2979	2418	1151	2511
- 1970	2949	2026	833	2542
Commune	Chincolco	Petorca		
Civil Registration District	Chincolco	Petorca	Hierro Viejo	
Area (square kilometers)	589	186	792	
Dates of Existence	1895- (dismembered from Petorca)	1885-	1885-1927 (Annexed to Petorca)	
Census Districts (Pop. 1970)	Pedernal 184			Pedegua 987
	Chalaco 478			Artificio 694
	Sobrante 564			Las Palmas 861
	Chincolco 1923			

Sources: INE, Anuario Estadistico, vol. 3: Politica y Administracion (Santiago, 1919), p. 8. Espinosa, pp. 157-164. Archivo de la Intendencia de Aconcagua (San Felipe) unpublished maps and instructions for 1940 and 1952 censuses (uncatalogued, untitled, not paginated). 1970 data supplied by INE from manuscripts. See also successive census publications 1813-1952.

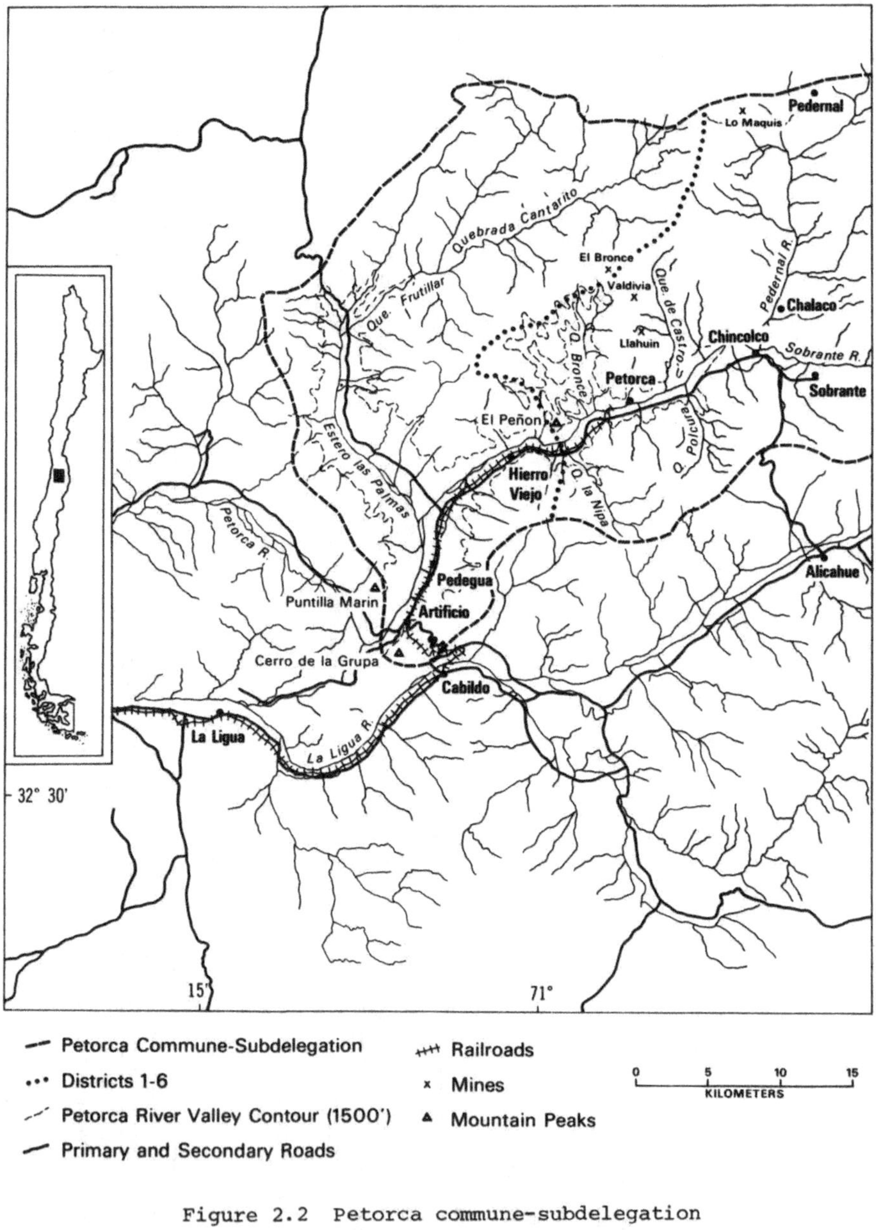

Figure 2.2 Petorca commune-subdelegation

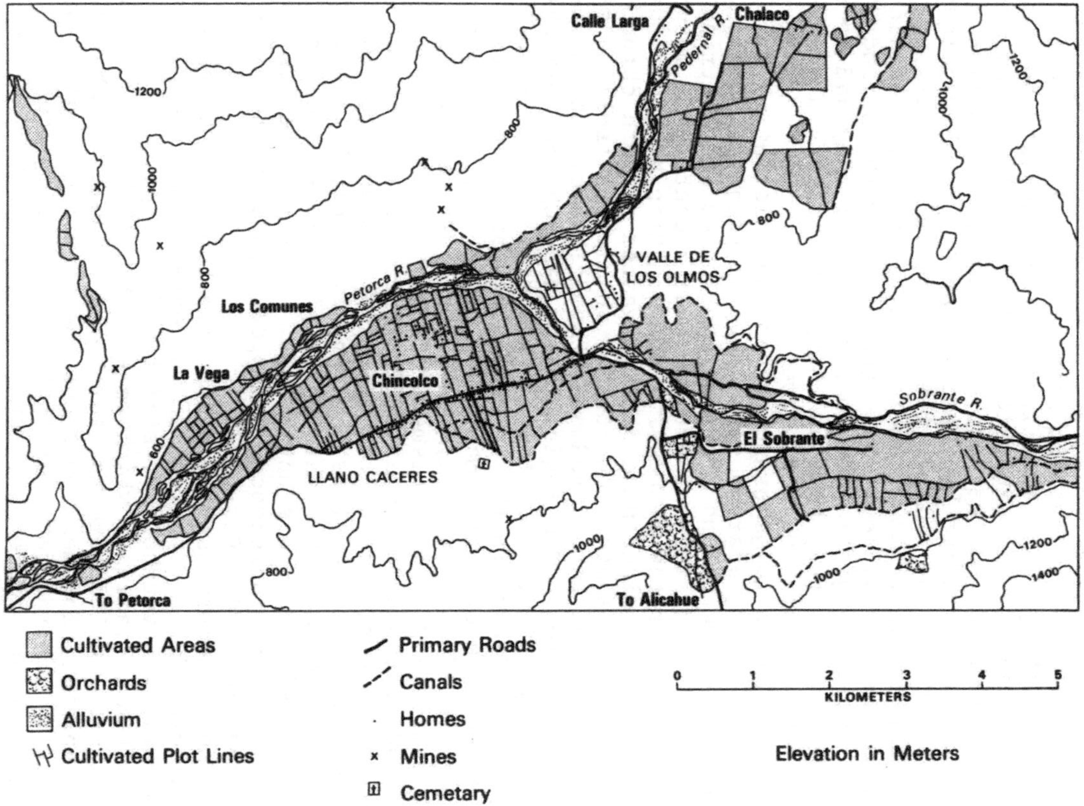

Figure 2.3 Cultivation patterns in Chincolco, ca. 1955

retained its dimensions as laid out two centuries ago: a strip four blocks wide and about twenty long. The most dispersed settlements occur in the ravines and gulches of the Western extreme of the valley (Cantarito, Frutillar, and Las Palmas). Moreover, if hamlets have built up at Artificio and around the old hacienda houses at Pedegua, these settlements are some twenty kilometers from the Petorca civil registry office, the parish church, and the hospital. Once La Grupa tunnel was completed at the turn of the century, services for people living in the western section of the parish were closer at hand across the mountain at Cabildo. The exclusion of families living at Artificio, Pedegua, Las Palmas, Cantarito, and Frutillar seem further justified by their distance from the administrative seat of the valley, their dispersed population, and their proximity to an evermore dynamic, fully serviced town in the next valley. Nevertheless, for the period of ecclesiastical registration (prior to 1885) they had to be included in the study because the parish priests did not regularly note precise residences.

In addition to geographical and administrative criteria for selecting a study site, several technical and substantive considerations are important as well. A string of well-kept registers stretching over a century or more is essential for the successful construction of genealogical histories. Since much data is wasted at both chronological ends of a study because of incomplete family histories, a longer period reduces proportionately the unusable genealogies. The registers for many Chilean parishes show highly erratic registration patterns as late as 1860.[9] The first baptisms in the Petorca books are dated 1728, but no entries exist for marriages prior to 1767 or burials before 1768. Moreover, the records are erratically kept until 1838. No baptisms are found for the period August 1803 through September 1807. Few marriage entries survive for the years of the wars for independence; the Petorca marriage registers show an almost total absence of marriages from May 1816 through April 1824, and do not achieve credible levels until 1838. Burial registers attain a certain consistency--as opposed to completeness--from the mid-1830s (Figure 2.4).

The procedure used here has been to construct family genealogies for all periods to the extent that the registers permit; nevertheless, strictly demographic analysis is limited to families which began after 1839. The family genealogies include events registered through December 31, 1970; however, for most purposes the termination date for presently existing families is April 22, 1970, the date of the most recent national census. Since the usual criteria for establishing the presence of families, the death of one of the spouses, is impossible to apply to young, currently extant families, the list of inhabitants made in 1970 cap off their histories. Aggregate registration data has been collected through March 15, 1977 and are used to

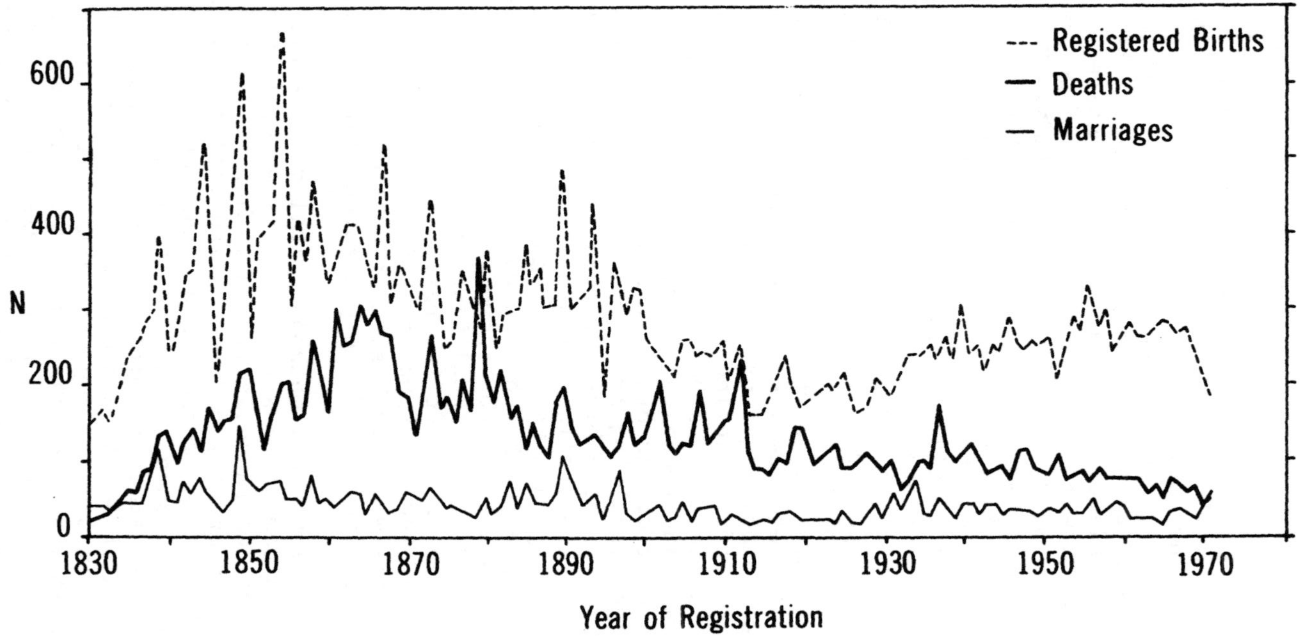

Figure 2.4 Marriages, deaths, and registered births for study area: 1830-1970

extend demographic interpretation through the mid-1970s.

Large populations make the construction of family genealogies excessively arduous. The method, developed to its most sophisticated level by French historical demographers, consists of the extraction of all registered births, deaths, and marriages (or more precisely, baptisms, burials, and marriages) from registry books.[10] In this instance over 100,000 entries were copied and then linked to make up the family genealogies.

Given the chronological span of the study and the data requirements, a rural community with a rather stagnant demographic history was the inevitable choice. Communities which grew to town or city size would be too large and their populations too mobile for study. On the other hand districts with moderate increases would not have maintained their territorial or registrational integrity over the span of the century. This methodological restriction still left a field of several score parishes as potential candidates. The population of many hamlets within the Chilean Central Valley have increased hardly at all over the past century. It should also be apparent that this peculiar requirement has significant substantive implications. The community must have been pressing against its resources, or at least relative to other local economies, expelling a greater share of its native-born population and attracting relatively fewer migrants.

The presence of a hospital was also a significant substantive and technical consideration. During recent decades, most births occur in hospitals; therefore, to reduce biases resulting from women temporarily leaving their communities to give birth, it was essential to select a study area with a clinic within its administrative limits. Moreover, hospitals have been important agents of demographic change in the Chilean countryside, both in improving infant mortality and reducing fertility. Rural communities with health facilities are not the exception in Chile. Since the 1880s the national government has actively supported the construction and maintenance of clinics. In 1925 there were 119 hospitals scattered throughout the Republic, an average of one per three registration districts.[11]

In summary then, methodological constraints force one to select a community with well-defined administrative and geographical characteristics, a rather stagnant local economy, and stable, moderate-sized population. Atypicality should not be considered a hindrance to scientific analysis. Any specific community can never be considered typical of a national aggregate. Each community has its own particular social and economic dynamics which distinguish it from others, apparent similarities in size, structure, or economy notwithstanding. If methodological considerations predominated in the selection of a study site, it was with a conviction that, whatever the choice, generalizations could be developed only through an imaginative understanding of the demographic and social dynamics of the community and not by misguided confidence in its typicality or the mechanical application of statistical formula.

The Chilean countryside is literally covered by demographic and economically stagnant communities. Most reached their apogee by 1875 and many have hardly expanded since. With land tenure patterns having been firmly established shortly after the Spanish conquest, with large landowners refusing to permit the work force to expand onto large estates, and with small plots shattering to a level of bare minimum subsistence, the countryside has expelled the bulk of its potential natural increase for well over a century. The demographic evolution of Petorca was not exceptional in this respect. Putaendo, Catemu, Calle Larga, Casablanca, El Monte, Alhué, Mostazal, Doñihue, Coltauco, Pichidegua, Olivar, Malloa, Chépica--all are communes located in central valley provinces (Aconcagua to Colchagua) which experienced virtually no increase in population size from 1875 to 1952.[12] The principal population clusters in Central Chile to expand in this period were cities--trade, communication, and administrative centers offering social and economic opportunities unavailable in the countryside.

For generations, land tenure patterns were important determinants of population flows in rural Chile. Spanish land grants dating in many instances from the mid-sixteenth century favored large holdings. If the process of land ownership and the formation of great estates was much more dynamic than the hoary images pictured in the history books of an earlier generation--families ruling their latifundia from generation to generation--in the main, a binary system of land ownership dominated the Chilean countryside. A few rich and powerful families established a monopoly over most of the occupied territory. Poorer families owned rights only to miniscule strips of lands. Notwithstanding the exceptional fertility and the intensive cultivation characteristic of the microplots, by 1875, many were no longer capable of providing a patrimony for succeeding generations. The lands of the great estates were usually unavailable to the small holders. The latifundia often changed ownership, but generally they were sold in their entirety. Large landowners allowed access only to a necessary and privileged few <u>inquilinos</u>, or sharecroppers, who were granted land and grazing rights in exchange for supplying the labor needs of the estate. This exchange often made the inquilinos into labor brokers who recruited family, friends, or vagabonds from a neighboring village to help with planting and harvesting or branding and roundup. Denied a secure access to land and proffered only sporadic employment, most of these casual laborers, both female and male, were forced to strike out at a young age seeking employment elsewhere--in nitrate and copper mines, on the southern agricultural frontier, and mostly in the rapidly growing cities. The countryfolk who stayed were usually those with a promise of land rights, with less ambition, or perhaps with stronger family ties. Nevertheless, from 1875 to 1952 rural populations in the Central Valley hardly increased.[13]

THE SETTLING OF PETORCA

The evolution of property rights and settlement patterns in the Petorca Valley is remarkably similar to the developments which have been documented for a contiguous valley, the Putaendo, and the Valle del Puangue near Santiago. The story for Petorca differs only in minor details. In 1591 Captain Ernando Somero Gallegos de Andrade was granted the entire Petorca Valley "with all its unoccupied lands" from the mouth of the Petorca River to its uppermost headwaters in "the snow-covered mountains."[14] Unlike the histories of Putaendo or Puangue, the titles to Petorca Valley underwent only a single change over the following century and a half. In 1606, the lands were transferred to the Augustine Convent and the entire expanse remained under their control until the founding of Petorca in 1780. If ownership by a religious corporation was unusual in Chile, this affiliation did not affect eventual settlement patterns in the Petorca Valley. Many towns were founded in Chile in the eighteenth century, and distributions of farms and townsites were based on criteria of wealth and character understood by both rich and poor. Settlers were alloted plots according to their abilities to found and maintain a settlement, facts explicitly recognized in the census enumerations carried out to establish allotment rights. The Convent was able to delay the final distributions for over twenty-five years (1753-1780) through litigation to ensure that the new title holders would provide recompense for the lost lands either through an immediate cash payment or an annual nonredeeming mortgage (censo).[15]

Unlike many other Chilean villages founded at this time, allocations for Petorca included extensive agricultural and grazing lands as well. The settlers convinced the Royal Commission on Population to force the Convent to make lands available for gardens, farms, and ranches. Consequently, lands stretching from El Peñon to the Alicahue Road, and including all the intermediate ravines draining into the river and the mountainsides as well, were assigned to settlers or set aside for village commons.[16]

The roots of the maldistribution of lands, antedating the initial division, were firmly planted in the final allotments of 1780. A handful of families were awarded very large tracts, while most settlers obtained a simple village plot barely sufficient for constructing a house and a small garden. The allotments legitimatized occupation rights established days to decades earlier (based on rental agreements with the Augustines).

"For being one of the principal and oldest settlers whose notorious merits is known by everyone and for the considerable sums he expended on the affairs of the settlement and pursuing the suits [against the Convent] which have presented themselves,"[17] Don Matias Cáceres received seven awards: a townsite, a farm, two plots with ore-grinding mills, and three ranches suitable for livestock. The grant totaled almost two thousand pesos or 18.8 percent of all awards by value. Several of Don Matias' sons also received town lots. Don Jose Sepúlveda received only six awards, but the value of his grants exceeded even those of the Cáceres--30.8 percent of the total.[18]

POPULATION, LAND, AND POLITICS

Juridical and economic realities determined the division of rural properties into large estates and modest farms. Subsequent demographic developments shattered the farms into literally hundreds of microplots while the huge ranches and farms retained their original integrity. Only the wealthiest were able to avoid the effects of Spanish inheritance laws which mandated equal division amongst all legitimate heirs (save a portion at the free disposition of the testator).[19] For small property holders lacking other assets, their farms had to be split into increasingly smaller fragments. Eventually the sections became too tiny to provide a livelihood for the heirs. Aware that the family offered few opportunities, offspring were forced to leave the homestead. By the 1830s the notarial records contain frequent references to the disposal of inheritances of people of unknown whereabouts.[20]

Impoverishment through generational succession was a fate experienced not only by the small holders. All families who remained for more than a generation and restricted their economic assets to enterprises in the valley suffered a similar fate. The richest families either moved on with the second generation or became impoverished as well. The history of the Cáceres family is perhaps the most extreme example of a process repeated many times by relatively accommodated families whose economic and social position collapsed with succeeding generations.

Matias Cáceres married Petronila Agredo in 1743 and both immediately embarked on highly productive careers--he, as a miner; she, as wife and mother. Over the following twenty-six years, Doña Petronila bore twenty-one children (and apparently died in childbirth), while Don Matias made a fortune in mining. They were unable to transmit their good fortune to their children. Eleven died at young ages; five daughters married and left the village. Only one of the sons married and remained at the homestead. Five years after his wife's death Don Matias remarried, at age 53, and had eight children by his second wife, Doña

Ana Josefa Pastén. The estate began to disintegrate immediately upon his death in 1791. To satisfy the claims of his children, one townsite and both ore mills (valued at $5,000) were sold. The following year the livestock ranches were disposed of to satisfy back interest due the Augustines. Over the next forty years Doña Ana administered the gradual dismemberment of the remnants of the estate. According to the tax assessments of 1834, less than ten cuadras remained valued at $150. The children of the second marriage had received only $122 each as their shares of the inheritance. The clan was reduced to two sons and one daughter who continued to farm the family holdings in Llano Cáceres (see Figure 2.3), although relations between children of the two marriages led to at least one lawsuit. In the 1870s, after decades of rising land values, Cáceres heirs owned properties valued at $368 consisting of five hijuelas and one small plot yet to be divided among five others. Two of Don Matias' grandsons, now reduced to poverty, repeatedly borrowed seeds from the public granary to sow their crops on strips valued at only 60 to 75 pesos each.[21]

If Don Matias had been alive to survey property titles in 1870 he would have immediately recognized all of the great estates, but most of the family names of the largest holdings would have surprised him. Pedernal, Frutillar, Pedegua, La Ñipa, Durazno, El Sobrante--all the major holdings continued as integral properties, just as he had known them two generations earlier. However, he would have been astonished by the explosion in the number of small properties achieved with no threat or expense to the boundaries of the large estates and ranches. He would have been shocked by the impoverishment of some of the great families, including his own, and the disappearance of others. No more than a handful of their descendants remained and most of these were spinsters or bachelors living on solitary townsites. Sepúlveda, Murúa, Montt, Prado, Umeres--all were great and powerful families known to Don Matias, but who, over the decades, departed the valley and ridded themselves of their holdings there, seeking to maintain or expand their fortunes in enterprises more profitable than Petorca's fickle mines and barren soils. However, the changes were more apparent than real. The elites were only circulating. The Silvas intermarried with and replaced the Sepúlvedas, the Montts and Prados, with the Larraíns. To be sure these families were known to Don Matias, but they were not the most important settlers in his day. They had been active in mining and several were important merchants, but they had not been the principal settlers.[22]

The highly skewed land tenure patterns not only persisted, but intensified as the poorer families were forced to divide their sole assets. Meanwhile the rich families, such as the Cáceres, when pushed to the extreme sold their large holdings as a unit with the stables, tools, irrigation ditches, and pastures intact to fetch a premium price.

Only the richest families with the most diversified interests could avoid the inevitable decline demanded by inexorable demographic and social forces. The moderate size holdings still remaining in the 1830s had virtually disappeared by 1874 (Figure 2.5). In 1833, the upper-middle property holders (those in the 60-90 percentiles) owned 32 percent of the land (by value). Forty-five years later the same group owned only 14 percent. Meanwhile, the upper 10 percentile increased its share from 45 to more than 75 percent. The small holders, the share of land owned by the bottom 50 percentile, hardly changed at all (7.5 percent to 7 percent).[23]

Borde and Góngora document a similar process in the Puangue Valley.[24] Baraona and others discovered similar developments in Putaendo.[25] Bauer has recently demonstrated similar patterns for much of the Chilean Central Valley.[26] Land tenure patterns, rooted in the colonial past and virtually unchanged in the face of an expanding population and growing agricultural markets, literally expelled young men from the countryside. Political defiance was unorganized, marginal, and individualized. A peasant might illegally occupy a strip of unguarded land in some obscure nook of a vast estate, but there was no challenge to the legitimacy of land rights nor demands for a more equitable distribution of land.

These developments were not restrained by the wars of independence or the founding of the Republic. During the Independence struggles, Republican leaders used their authority to favor their supporters, which tended to prejudice the well being of the small holders. This favoritism is demonstrated in the leaders' relations with the Augustine Convent and settlers. For over seventy years the Convent had intermittently filed suits against the settlers. Many ended in stalemate; others, after lengthy appeals, ordered the settlers to reach an agreement to pay often heavily discounted overdue interest. Nevertheless, the power of the state had been used sparingly, the courts paid strict attention to law, and the final rulings were impartial.[27] The concerns of revolutionary leaders were those of winning a war and not justice. In 1818, when the Augustines brought a suit against the settlers to force the payment of accounts past due and offered half of the proceeds to the Republican cause for the purchase of rifles, the local governor was ordered to collect the accounts in arrears forthwith and remit half to the revolutionary authorities.[28] The following year, when special taxes were levied, many of the wealthiest property holders (e.g. Don Santiago Larraín, Don José Nicolas de la Serda, Don José Manuel Irrarazával, Don Romualdo Silva, etc.) used their connections to obtain dispensations. Whatever the Republic governor collected came from the small holders.[29]

After Independence was won, an ungraduated land tax

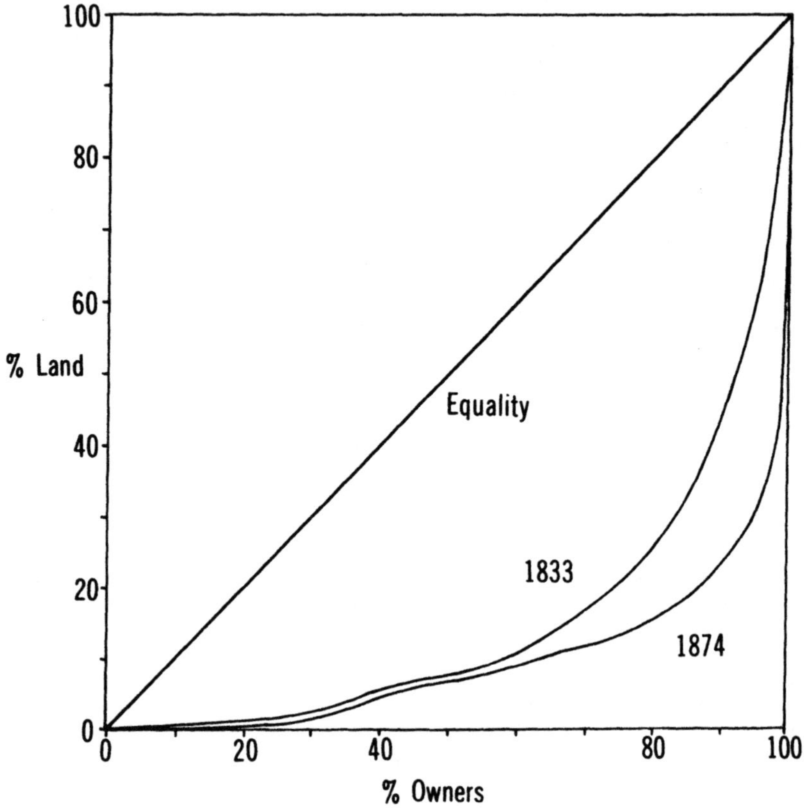

Sources: Tax evaluations for 1833, 1874-1878. See Note 23.

Figure 2.5 Growing inequality of land holdings: Petorca, 1833, 1874

was enacted and on several occasions consideration was given to extending it to the tiniest holders (those with property worth less than twenty-five pesos) to force them to pay their fair share of taxes and encourage them to produce for the market.[30] Legislative reforms to provide land for the landless never went beyond exhortations to the latifundistas to accept more sharecroppers and thereby permit more intensive cultivation of their very extensive estates.[31] Land titles remained sacrosanct. The small peasantry was at the mercy of inexorable economic and demographic processes reinforced by unchallenged juridical principles.

Unrelieved poverty or the abandonment of family were the principal alternatives facing young men in rural Chile. The population data show that for more than a century the overwhelming response in one parish after another throughout the Central Valley has been to migrate.[32] Within the Petorca Valley whenever bits of large estates were sold off (as happened with a portion of Pedegua in 1876)[33] or new villages founded (Hierro Viejo in the 1850s)[34] the results were shortlived; within a generation the problem of insufficient land revived with its accustomed force.

The number of agricultural property holders in the Petorca Valley more than doubled from 1833 to 1878 (67 to 184). Over the next half century they tripled (647 in 1935) and then increased very slightly to 1964 (835).[35] In the last decade pressure for agrarian reform has been overwhelming. All the large fundos in the valley were expropriated and distributed to peasant cooperatives. In 1974 the process was halted, reversed, and aggravated by the land policies of the military Junta.[36] Regardless of the Junta's eventual land program, the outlook for any reduction in the rate of expulsion of population from the countryside appears dim (unless the Junta's economic policies destroy the urban economy in the long run as well as the short). Even with a tremendous decline in fertility apparent since the mid-1960s, the migration patterns of the past will persist. While data were being collected for this study (1970-1971, 1977), farmers repeatedly related their need to keep their families small in order to provide remunerative work for their children. Nevertheless their families continue to exceed the available economic opportunities given present economic, social, and political conditions.

THE MINES OF PETORCA

> This department the richest [in mining] some years back, principally in gold for it surpassed all the others in the Republic because of its rich output, is now in a state of total prostration. The largest part of its mines are

> completely abandoned, some full of water, others destroyed and others in need of long shafts to make them productive . . . .
>
> Annual Report of the Governor of Petorca, March, 1886

If most other rural districts in the Central Valley are solely dependent on the soil, Petorca has always had an additional resource: minerals. However, the mines of the Norte Chico have challenged the ingenuity and exhausted the wealth of several generations. In fact, much of the fame of Petorca Valley's ancient mines is relative rather than absolute. Their greatness shines only in comparison to the total impoverishment of most other Chilean settlements in the colonial era. As late as 1813 Petorca was larger than many communities which today rank as major regional cities.[37] In 1813, Petorca was about the same size as San Felipe, Los Andes, and La Ligua. It ranked closely behind Quillota and Copiapó. In terms of population size even La Serena and Valparaiso, notwithstanding their much older origins, were only just twice as large as Petorca (5500 versus 2800); by 1960 they had grown to 50,000 and 250,000, respectively, while the population of Petorca had declined to 2000. The principal reason for Petorca's earlier growth was gold; the major cause for the community's decline was a lack of it. In 1813, the Petorca Valley (from El Sobrante to Puntilla Marin) accounted for 1.9 percent of the population of the Bishopric of Santiago (from the Rio Maule to Coquimbo Province), but over 14 percent of all miners and over 5 percent of the merchants were enumerated in the Petorca Valley.[38] For over a century its mountains had grudgingly yielded precious metals to those with the tenacity to dig for them, with the capital to withstand months and even years of mining nothing but worthless rock, and with the luck to find them.

Given the scarce resources and desperate situation of most of the miners and the difficulty of extracting the ore, Petorca's mines were never properly exploited. They always seem to have been in a state of decay, even from the first major, prolonged strikes in the 1720s. One of the earliest surviving law suits to take place in the valley (1728) stemmed from the collapse of a mine shaft because of improper diggings (incidentally, on a claim worked by Don Matias' father).[39] Invariably, when a shaft appeared to have been exhausted, or perhaps when the mine owner's personal finances reached a crisis, the diggings were destroyed by mining the pillars and arches which had been constructed to sustain the shaft. After the mine was abandoned, another miner with greater faith, fewer debts, or perhaps more desperation would put a crew in the destroyed shafts and try to rebuild sufficiently to permit mining to proceed.[40] By 1730 an examiner reported what was to become a litany repeated by all those who came after him:

> The mine Nuestra Senora del Rosario, 15 marks [estados] deep. There are no bridges although there should be seven. There are small pillars twenty yards long and all of them together would amount to less than four cargas. There is a lot of stone.
>
> Santa Cruz Mine, 25 marks deep with not a single bridge although it should have twelve two yards thick. The mine is dangerous and could be worked only at great cost.[41]

Spanish mining laws, designed to ensure safety and maximum benefit for the Crown, served for naught in the face of the daily exigencies under which Petorcan miners operated.

Three-quarters of a century later the economic realities of gold mining in Petorca had not changed even though the mines were producing as never before. According to an inspection made in January 1800, thirteen claims in the district were producing over $60,000 per year plus an estimated $30,000 which escaped reporting. Nevertheless, there were some 600 shafts which had been "despoiled, destroyed and abandoned."[42] The last decades of Spanish rule were probably the richest in the valley's history. Certainly the number of homicides and robberies were greater at this time than at any other.[43] On the founding of a notary office in 1792, a town father dryly observed that the office should be worth only $300 a year "because the misery and poverty of most of the valley's inhabitants, dedicated to working mines, only produced drunkenness, petty suits and homocides" rather than more remunerative litigations, public instruments, embargos, commissions, etc.[44] In those years the village's inhabitants consumed 250 liters of wine and 100 liters of aguardiente daily (at least, taxes were paid on that amount), which averages out to about one-half liter per day per adult male.[45] The auction of the concession for the annual festival day often went for more than 300 pesos.[46] By 1830 the transition from colony to republic was complete; for Petorcans the mining boom had collapsed. In 1833 the auction of all the village's monopolies produced the miserable sum of fifty pesos.[47]

Why the decadence? Probably the most important fact was not that Petorca or its mines had changed, but that the larger economy of which it was a part had grown and become more dynamic. Petorca's mines were no longer attractive when compared with the silver bonanzas of Arqueros (discovered in 1825) and Chañarcillo (1832).[48] Although poorer miners stayed on in the valley, the great merchants, who had always financed most of the mining operations and ended up with most of the profits, left Petorca in search of more favorable investments. The once attractive shafts were abandoned to solitary scavengers.

Some large operations continued, but they were only of marginal benefit, employing at most several score workers. At least one operation shifted to copper mining and adopted new refining technology, the reverberatory furnace, but the results were disappointing in the face of Petorca's woefully inadequate roads and fuel supplies.[49] Once the woods were exhausted, the operation folded. A general survey made in 1886 found sixteen tiny operations only half of which made any profits for their owners. Fewer than two hundred workers were employed in mining, where almost six hundred had worked in 1813.[50] In 1894 the editors of the local newspaper ruefully observed:

> The mining industry, once the lifeblood of the village, is now worked on such a small scale that it is not a vital and progressive industry but a simple game of chance in which the poor fearfully sacrifice their savings and the rich in the notion that chance will favor them, throw a few coins to the ground, hoping that they will multiply themselves.[51]

Nor did the situation change in the twentieth century. The economic census of 1943 found 329 miners working thirty-two separate operations. Five copper works employed only twenty-three men. Most mined the now ancient diggings at El Bronce.[52] The revaluation of gold after the Great Depression made the old mines profitable again, although actual methods continued to be woefully antiquated and under-capitalized. Virtually no machinery was used; donkeys and mules carried out the ores. In every economic depression young Petorcans take their picks and strike out for the mines, as occurred again after September 1973. With a donkey, simple tools, perhaps a bit of powder, and much luck, they find enough gold to keep their families in necessities.

In 1970 there were only 177 miners working in the valley east of El Peñon. The largest camp had forty-five miners and used pneumatic drills, explosives, and modern refining techniques to extract copper. A half dozen other mines employed between five and fifteen men. The bulk of the miners continued the tradition of marginal mining as an almost solitary pursuit.[53] Most advances in mining technology made the mines in the Petorca Valley unattractive. The ores were too limited to justify the major capital investments required to exploit them in competition with even the small copper mining operations of the Norte Chico. Although two or three copper mines have been modernized, new techniques acquired, capital invested, and the latest refining methods applied, the benefits for the valley have been almost casual and indirect. The mining companies are formed by outsiders who obtain most of their supplies directly from wholesalers in Valparaiso and Santiago.[54] Many of the mine workers are from outside the valley as well.[55] Consequently, the economic impact of the heavily capitalized operations for the community is reduced.

A STATIC POPULATION

> The day will come when it will be difficult even for public employees to earn a living in Petorca.
>
> Voz de Petorca, September 23, 1894

With the collapse of mining and stagnation of agriculture, public administration became one of the means for maintaining a certain level of economic vitality in the community. As a result of the political reorganization of 1830, Petorca was selected as the gubernatorial seat for the northern sector of Aconcagua Province, Petorca Department. However, its economic decadence and poor geographical location eventually robbed the community of administrative pretensions. The local elite fought a tenacious battle over many generations to maintain through political persuasion what had been lost through economic and geopolitical realities.[56] Finally, in 1936, the inevitable ignominy was suffered. Petorca Department was merged with its neighbor, La Ligua, and while the new department retained the historic name, government offices were moved to La Ligua--a final judgment on the lowly economic and political status of Petorca Village.[57]

Thenceforth, public employment for Petorcans would be confined to service, as opposed to administrative, jobs: teaching, nursing, and construction. In 1970 there were 112 people on the public payrolls; exactly one-half worked on highway maintenance ("vialidad")![58] The contribution of public employment as a source of cash income should not be underestimated. Most public employees were native to the community and resided with their families. Only the more prestigious and remunerative positions, such as teachers, doctors, and policemen, were held by outsiders, many of whom were unmarried or not living with their families.

Table 2.2 summarizes the global population trends of the valley according to the official censuses. The figures indicate much greater fluctuations than probably took place. Because of the unsettled conditions during the independence wars, the 1813 census probably had a relatively larger undercount than later censuses. The population peaks of 1885 and 1907 seem to be the result of fraud. In both instances, it appears that counts for districts in Chincolco were inflated, probably for electoral purposes.[59] All of the "increases" for those years occurred in district two while district three shows slight declines. Thus, we may conclude that the total population of the valley has remained very stable over a century or more. The gradual increase to approximately 10,000 inhabitants in 1865 was followed by a gentle, prolonged decline to 6,600 in 1930 and a slow recovery to 8,500 in 1952.

If the economic history of the Petorca Valley is a depressing one, it is not exceptional. What makes Petorca different from other rural communities in Central Chile is that it experienced a gold rush, an era of prosperity that

TABLE 2.2
Population of Petorca Parish, 1813-1970

Census Year	Total Population	Average Annual Intercensal Change
1813	5712	
1845	7325	0.8%
1854	7989	0.8
1865	9576	1.7
1875	9270	-0.3
1885	11814	2.4
1895	7423	-4.6
1907	14036	5.3
1920	7304	-5.0
1930	6572	-1.1
1940	7825	1.8
1952	8408	0.6
1960	8465	0.1
1970	8350	-0.1
1813-1865		0.8
1865-1930		-0.6
1930-1970		0.6

Sources: Official censuses. 1970 figures provided by the Census Bureau from manuscript data.

vanished long ago. For generations now Petorcans have struggled within the same kinds of social and economic constraints suffered by the people of Putaendo and Puangue, Catemu and Coltauco.

Since the middle of the nineteenth century Petorcans (and probably Chilean country-folk in general) have shown an amazing demographic flexibility in dealing with difficult economic and social circumstances. Confronted with horrifying epidemics, they struggled to build hospitals and to keep them stocked with medicines. Recognizing the mortiferous effects of their polluted water supplies, they built a sanitary water system with very limited means and often their own hands. When faced with contracting economic opportunities, some delayed marriage and others forsook marriage completely. The bulk of each generation abandoned their homes to seek a more generous livelihood elsewhere. Finally the present generation, encountering a demographic revolution the intensity and pace of which few peoples of any historical epoch have ever known, quickly and effectively reduced their fertility to maintain a parity between their economic circumstances and the size of their families.

NOTES

1. Voz de Petorca; April 8, 1894, August 5, 1894, September 23, 1894, September 6, 1908, December 2, 1906, March 6, 1904. Governors' reports and communications: GP, 1846; GP, 1871; GP, 1874-78; GP, 1877; GP, 1885, GP, 1900. The Archivo de la Intendencia de Aconcagua in San Felipe is unorganized. Volumes are identified by a stamp on the spine (e.g. "Gobernación de Petorca, 1874-78") and are unpaginated.

2. Carlos Keller R., "Diccionario Económico-geográfico de la Republica de Chile," unpublished manuscript, pp. 1-6. Enrique Espinosa, Jeografía descriptiva de la República de Chile, 4th ed. (Santiago, 1897), pp. 156-164.

3. Keller, "Diccionario Económico-geográfico," pp. 2, 10. Corporación de Fomento de la Producción, (CORFO), Geografía económica de Chile, rev. ed. (Santiago, 1967), pp. 16-17 and 168-169.

4. Keller, "Diccionario Económico-geográfico," pp. 23-35. CORFO, Geografía económica, pp. 208-210, 242-243. For reports, contracts, and litigation over the cutting of wood for the refineries see: JP, vol. 1, pieza 7 (1833-1841); NP, vol. 49, f. 71 (1875), MI, vol. 317 (1855), and GP, 1875.

5. See GP, 1846, 1871, 1874-78, 1877, 1900; Voz de Petorca, August 5, 1894, March 19, 1905 has extensive reports; most issues lament the poor roads which link the department with the rest of the country.

6. For the founding documents see CPGEN, vol. 938, legajo 17029; and FV, vol. 918. The laws dealing with boundary changes for Aconcagua Province are noted in Servicio Nacional de Estadistica y Censos (INE), XII Censo general de población y I de vivienda, vol. 3: Nucleo Central I (Santiago, 1952), pp. v-vi.

7. FV, vol. 918.

8. Keller, "Diccionario Económico-geográfico," pp. 1-9, gives precise figures for census districts. See also the excellent series of maps scale 1:50,000 by the Instituto Geográfico Militar de Chile, first edition, (Santiago, 1968), map numbers 3145-7100 through 3215-7030, based on airphotos and classifications made 1954-1959.

9. The Anuario estadístico, primera entrega (Santiago, 1860) lists baptisms, marriages, and burials for each parish from 1848 through 1858. Data for subsequent years are published intermittently. The Archives Division of the Central Civil Registry Office maintains a manuscript tabulation for each registration district from its founding.

10. Michel Fleury and Louis Henry, Noveau manuel de dépouillement et d'exploitation de l'état civil ancién (Paris, 1965), pp. 118-162. The quality of Chilean registers are exceptionally poor in comparison to those of French parishes in the eighteenth century. For a discussion of data quality and procedures used in this study, see Appendix I.

11. INE, Annuario estadístico de la República de Chile, vol. 2: Beneficiencia, medicina e higiene, 1925, p. 5.

12. INE, Censo de . . . 1952, vol. 3, pp. xvi-xxxi.

13. Ibid.

14. FV, vol. 918, f. 84-103.

15. CPGEN, legajos 1047, 1630, 3586, 17985, 18070, 18110, 18184 in vols. 223, 58, 92, 1015, 1024, 1028, 1032, respectively. See also

Archivo de la Provincia de los Agustinos, Escrituras, 1612-1895; and Fondo Antiguo (Archivo Nacional), vol. 2, pieza 1.

16. The surveys are presented in FV, vol. 918

17. Ibid.

18. Ibid.

19. Jean Borde y Mario Góngora, Evolución de la propiedad rural en el Valle del Puangue (Santiago, 1956), p. 54.

20. JP, vol. 8, pieza 19. NP, vol. 37, f. 51; vol. 39, f. 83; vol. 34, f. 16.

21. ANP, vol. 1, f. 16, f. 117; vol. 4, f. 197; vol. 9, f. 313; vol. 11, f. 7; vol. 3, f. 154, 204, 304, 348; vol. 4, f. 26, 114, 237, 250, 278, 295; vol. 6, f. 188; vol. 8, f. 9, 34, 39, 44, 132, 186, 215; vol. 9, f. 30; vol. 1881, f. 76; vol. 1890, f. 141. JP, vol. 4, pieza 12. MH, vol. 8, f. 164, 210-222. FV, vol. 918, f. 54, ff. Libro de Posito Pío, Archivo Parroquial de Petorca. Impuesto Agrícola. Rol de Contribuyentes (Lei de 18 de junio de 1874) vol. 1 (Valparaiso, 1875), Archivo Contaduría Mayor, Serie II, Catastro de Petorca 1834. GP, vol. 1874-78.

22. FV, vol. 918, f. 54, ff.

23. Derived from land cadasters collected for 1833 and 1874-1878. Usually these reports exclude the small plots from consideration but the Petorca returns seem to include plots of all sizes; some (all?) valued at only $12 are listed. See references in note 21 beginning with Impuesto Agrícola. The data for small properties in the 1870s are derived from manuscripts in GP and are added to the published individualized lists for the large farms in Impuesto Agrícola.

24. Borde and Góngora, Evolución de la, pp. 58-62, 83-87, 89-118.

25. Rafael Baraona, Ximena Aranda, and Roberto Santana, Valle de Putaendo: estudio de estructura agraria (Santiago, 1961), pp. 139-218.

26. Arnold J. Bauer, Chilean Rural Society from the Spanish Conquest to 1930 (Cambridge, England, 1975), pp. 117-144. Note that only one of the large estates was reduced in size by the partition process described by Bauer for La Companía (p. 131). The realities of farming and ranching in the arid Norte Chico may explain the persistence of the largest estancias.

27. See note 15.

28. JP, vol. 2, pieza 9. NP, vol. 5, unpaginated. MH, vol. 8, f. 164, ff. 189, ff.

29. MH, Ibid.

30. Bauer, Chilean Rural Society, p. 149.

31. See the curious proposal in MH, vol. 8, no page.

32. INE, Censo de . . . 1952, vol. 3, pp. xvi-xxi; vol. 4, pp. xvi-xx. Bauer, Chilean Rural Society, pp. 158-160. Carlos Hurtado Ruiz-Tagle, Concentración de la población y desarrollo económico: el caso chileno (Santiago, 1966), pp. 57-61.

33. NP, vol. 44, f. 8-12.

34. NP, vol. 34, f. 87, ff; vol. 48, f. 67-71. MI, vol. 317, f. 1, ff.

35. Catastro de Petorca 1834; Impuesto Agrícola . . . 1874; GP, vol. 1874-78; Keller, "Diccionario Económica-geográfico," p. 20. Keller's manuscript is an extraordinarily rich compilation of historical materials for the entire republic. Most recent conclusions are

based on the 1943 economic census carried out under his direction by the Ministerio de Hacienda. Only one volume on the Department of Arica was ever published. Water right controversies are not analyzed here--although they have been more important than land rights in the arid Norte Chico--because hard data on its distribution and use is difficult to find. A long history of suits between villagers and the fundo owners and miners is revealed in the various manuscript collections. See, for example, MI, Memoria Anual 1863, p. 29 and Voz de Petorca, August 11, 1908 for published snippets.

36. Conversations with peasants in March, 1977. At that time the Junta was considering distributing the large estates to individual holders. The peasants complained about a lack of voice in deciding who should receive lands and how they should be distributed. Agronomists in Santiago apparently made their decisions without consultations in the field.

37. Keller notes this in his manuscript, "Diccionario Económica-geográfico," p. 16.

38. Tabulated from the Censo de 1813.

39. CPGEN vol. 260, leg. 4052.

40. Fondo Antiguo (Archivo Nacional) vol. 34, pieza 1, f. 47.

41. CPGEN, vol. 232, leg. 3714.

42. NP, vol. 5, s/f.

43. See JP, vol. 15, pieza 77. Both the burial registers and the judicial archive are full of references to the violent life of the village toward the end of the colonial era.

44. CPGEN vol. 213, leg. 3442.

45. NP, vol. 5, s/f.

46. Real Audiencia (Archivo Nacional), vol. 563, pieza 4; JP vol. 7, legajo 4; NP, vol. 5, s/f.

47. Ibid.

48. Sergio Villalobos R., et al., Historia de Chile (Santiago, 1974), Vol. 3, pp. 414, 472-476.

49. See JP, vol. 1, legajo 7; MI, vol. 317; NP, vol. 49, f. 71; Keller, "Diccionario Económica-geográfico," p. 20.

50. Censo de 1813; and GP, 1886.

51. Voz de Petorca, September 23, 1894.

52. Keller, "Diccionario Económica-geográfico," p. 20, ff.

53. Tabulated from 1970 manuscript lists.

54. Conversations with local shopkeepers.

55. 1970 census manuscripts.

56. See for example MI, vol. 317, f. 28, 205; GP, 1895; Voz de Petorca, October 14, 1894; MH, vol. 8, f. 193-194.

57. Censo de . . . 1952, Nucleo central I, vol. 3, p. v.

58. The roads were being paved the day the census was taken; consequently, many farmers appeared as road workers (vialidad).

59. Keller ("Diccionario Económica-geográfico," pp. 10-19) develops this hypothesis with a detailed discussion.

3
Celibacy, Coupling, and Marriage

Marriage and the beginnings of family life have always constituted the most significant culturally determined transition in the lives of the people of the Petorca Valley. Much social life revolved around the rituals of courtship, concubinage, and marriage. Petorcans were willing to sacrifice several months' wages to marry. In the middle of the nineteenth century, when a day's work earned twenty-five centavos or less, laborers often paid the priest five pesos and even more to marry. Meanwhile, others sought companionship in concubinage. Celibacy was common, but not chastity. Sexual license and concubinage were conventional stages in courtship, often leading to marriage. The transitions were neither automatic nor inevitable. Marriage and family were determined as much by misery as morality.

Of all areas of family life, marriage has been the main concern of both the Catholic Church and the Chilean state. Typically marriage records are the most detailed, extensive, and complete. Often the village priest used six manuscript pages to record the details of marriage, while six births and as many as twenty deaths were inscribed on a single page. The personality of the vicar, his morals, social ideology, and administrative energy are revealed in the nuptial records or not at all. Likewise, ecclesiastical authorities often issued directives to the parish priests encouraging them to ensure that parishioners duly consecrate conjugal life and provide their offspring with the stable family life available only in marriage.

After 1885 with the declining authority of the priest and the cheapening of marriage by its conversion to a civil ceremony, fewer Petorcans wed, but concubinage rates rose to fill the void. Beginning in 1928 social rewards proffered by the state--social security, family allowances, and health care--were increasingly tied to having one's conjugal union lawfully inscribed. Consequently, in recent years marriage has become much more frequent and concubinage correspondingly less common. The timing of unions between men and women, a crucial social and demographic indicator, is conventionally ascertained by the age at marriage. However, given the customs of the people of Petorca with respect to premarital intercourse, it seems appropriate to use a complimentary measure as well, the age of coupling or pairing. Both provide insight into family initiation customs and demographic matters.

Until recent times permanent celibacy was a common state among adult Petorcans (Table 3.1). Approximately one out of four females born in the nineteenth century who lived beyond menopause did not marry. The celibacy rate for males was slightly lower (one in five), but the difference might be attributable to the relatively greater out-migration of single adult males. For those born before 1845, their lower rates may be due as much to juridical innovations as to changing patterns of family formation. With the institution of the civil registration system on January 1, 1885, official declarations of marital status required documentary proof rather than simple assertion. A sizeable minority of Petorcans, and Chileans in general, resisted the institution of civil marriage by marrying solely in the Church or not at all. Registrars, in accordance with civil law, responded by refusing to recognize Church marriages. Before the reforms of 1885 registration was in the hands of the parish priest, who often enjoyed a very brief tenure (averaging one-fifth that of a civil registrar) and administered a much larger territory (by 1895, Petorca parish had been split into three civil registration districts; see Table 2.1). Priests were unable to ascertain the marital status of the deceased as reliably as civil registrars. Lower celibacy rates for the earliest birth cohorts are not confirmed by the available census data (Table 3.2). The 1865 census manuscripts, the only check against the burial registers for people born before 1850, indicate much higher rates of permanent celibacy (30 percent compared to 21-22 percent). For later cohorts the death registration data are in broad agreement with census figures and indicate that roughly 30 percent of the female population never married. This general level is about 50 percent higher than the historical Western European marriage patterns. Recently, according to both census and vital registry data, celibacy rates in the Petorca Valley have declined sharply to less than 20 percent. In 1970, of ninety-nine women aged 50-59, only sixteen were single. The last cohort of women fully analyzable in the death inscriptions--those born during 1905-1909 and dying at ages 45-64--indicates a celibacy rate of 20 percent (N=15). The recent trend seems toward increased marriage rates.

THE CELIBATE ARE NOT CHASTE: NATURAL CHILDREN

Petorcans rarely confused celibacy with chastity.

TABLE 3.1
Permanent celibacy estimated from death registers

Decennial Birth Cohort	Celibate (%) Females Aged 45-64	Celibate (%) Males Aged 55-64	Deaths Females Aged 45-64	Deaths Males Aged 55-64
1825	21	17	82	60
1835	22	18	113	55
1845	30	27	104	49
1855	39	13	79	53
1865	19	37	68	30
1875	45	24	53	58
1885	26	13	46	31
1895	32	26	44	43
TOTAL	26	22	589	379

Dataset: Deaths

TABLE 3.2
Permanent celibacy estimated from census

Birth Cohort	Women Aged 50-59 Percent Single	Women Aged 50-59 N	Administrative Unit	Census
1806-1815	29.9	67	6 Districts	1865
1847-1856	32.3	944	Department	1907
1860-1869	29.4	717	Department	1920
1870-1879	30.5	226	Commune	1930
1905-1914	16.2	99	Study area	1970

Source: DP, Censo 1865; Censo de 1907, 291, 1305; Censo de 1920, 231, 243; Censo de 1930, 2:7, 53; 1970 Census manuscripts.

According to official inscriptions at least 30 percent of all births were born out of wedlock--politely referred to as "natural" children in the records (Table 3.3).[1] Nevertheless, legitimacy status at the time of registration is a misleading indicator of ultimate condition because many children were born in concubinage which later led to marriage. Births designated by the ultimate status of the child, as inferred from the family histories, indicate that real bastardy levels were 25-40 percent lower than

TABLE 3.3
Births by legitimacy status: Petorca, 1840-1969

	Legitimacy Status		
Birth Cohort	Legitimate (%)	Natural (%)	Total Births (N)
1840-1864	70.9	29.1	10,880
1865-1884	63.0	37.0	6,739
1885-1899	61.4	38.6	5,226
1900-1929	49.6	50.4	6,853
1930-1969	68.3	31.7	10,758

Dataset: All births

the conventional figures (Figure 3.1). The total proportion of births to mothers who ultimately married remained extraordinarily constant over time at slightly less than 60 percent. Because parish marriage inscriptions were included in the study through 1896, the rise in the proportion of natural children was delayed until the first decades of the twentieth century. During the period 1900-1929 popular lassitude toward civil sanction of conjugal unions produced a 50 percent increase in children born to mothers who ultimately married. At the same time the civil registrars' enforcement of stringent criteria for proving legitimacy and, to a certain extent, decreased migration into the valley, produced a substantial drop in legitimate children born to parents presumably married outside the valley. The trend in illegitimacy ratios reflects both changing family formation customs and registration innovations. The relative prevalence of concubinage is probably exaggerated by the figures for infants whose mothers were presumed never to have married. Increased out-migration in the twentieth century and declining adult mortality add further distortions. Nevertheless the basic level of bastardy has been high, and until 1930 the trend has always been upward. Lately the initial expenses of marriage have become trifling and no longer pose a monetary obstacle. At the same time the benefits from state-provided family allowances, unemployment compensation, and the like entice many from concubinage to marriage, reducing the proportion of illegitimate births to a historical low. Since 1950, the inferred bastardy ratio has fluctuated between 15 and 20 percent.

ILLICIT INTERCOURSE IN GOOD FAITH

Explanations of the relatively great incidence of

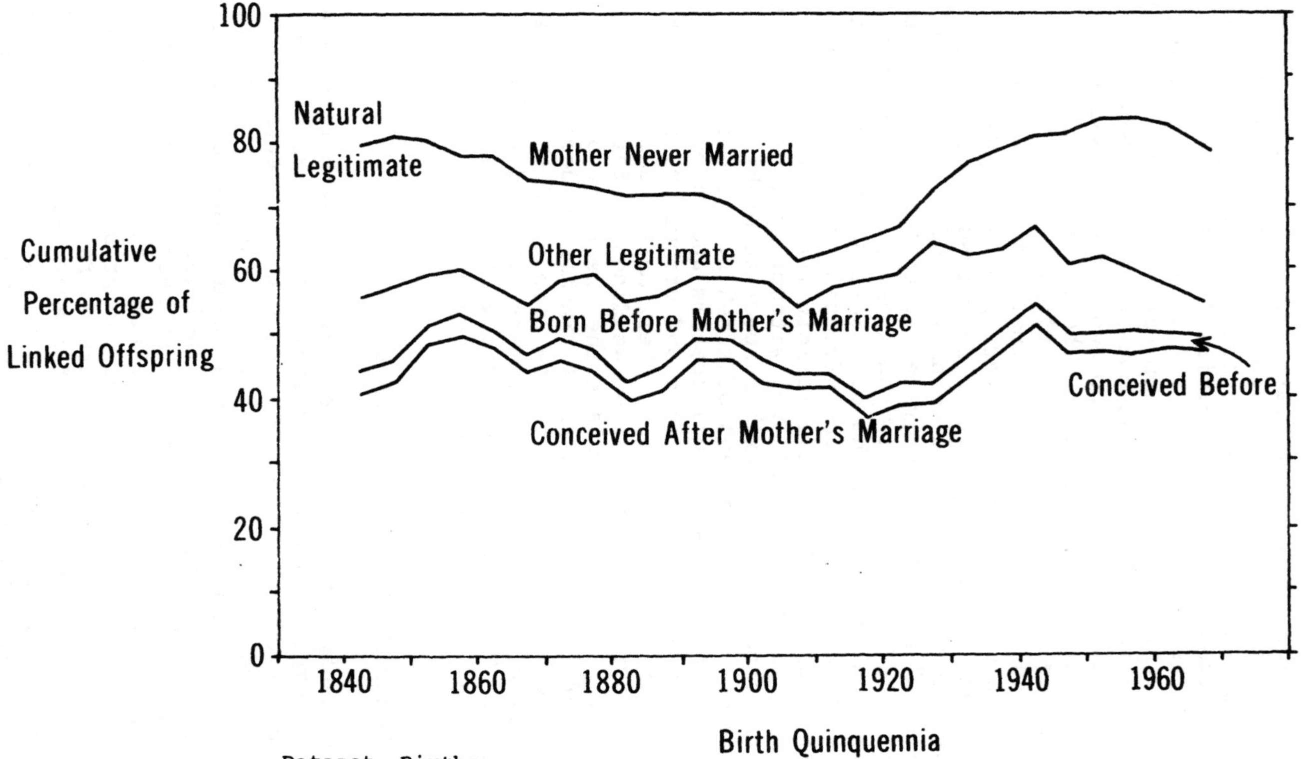

Dataset: Births

Figure 3.1 Petorca children by derived legitimacy status: 1840-1969

bastardy in Petorca Valley, and in the Norte Chico in general, reside in the economic misery of the zone coupled with an extraordinary degree of sexual passion, even promiscuity. The quantitative data cannot reveal the life pattern of sexual activity. Nevertheless, the marriage testimonies suggest that girls became sexually active in their mid-teens, while boys typically restrained themselves for several years longer. In 1848 a young bride of sixteen sought dispensation from canon law "for having had carnal relations with a first cousin of the groom," a day laborer of twenty-six years who swore that he was responsible for her pregnant state.[2] The pattern of sexual activity by age will be discussed below.

Courtship easily led to coitus, particularly if there was promise of marriage. Nor were promises always empty or inflated. In 1833 the vicar forwarded the solicitation of a mine foreman for the dispensation of an impediment to marriage. "Among the most grave causes that this unhappy man has cited, is that of having lived in illicit amity for five months and made the girl lose her honor with the promise of marriage." A not infrequent refrain in the nuptial records is that "the illicit intercourse was entered into in good faith," i.e. without knowledge that the union violated canon law with respect to prohibition of commerce within four degrees of kinship. Much of the analysis of premarital sexual customs and concubinage derives from statements of brides and grooms justifying the dispensation of impediments to their marriage (428 marriages, about 15 percent of the weddings performed from 1840-1894). Table 3.4 displays the frequency of impediments according to the degree of kinship as declared in the marriage records. Church law recognized three types of impediments--those by blood, marriage, and illicit intercourse. The degrees of kinship were determined by the generational distance between the espoused.[3]

THE WRETCHED STATE OF CONCUBINAGE

Courtship, concubinage, and marriage were intertwined, but in a complex fashion impossible to disentangle from the historical record. It is clear that the conception or birth of a child was cause for both advancing and retarding movement from one stage to another. The very desperate conditions of most Petorcan families discouraged their youth, particularly young men, from hastily entering marriage. The scarcity of housing, land, and even water subdued the desire for marriage and the pressing obligations of family, but not for sexual intercourse.

The extent and diversity of premarital sexual activity is frankly documented in the marriage testimonies. Although the records are silent about intercourse between non-kin, the frequency of premarital sexual relations was great indeed, if the accounts of dispensations of impediments

TABLE 3.4
Nuptial impediments according to degree of kinship, 1840-1894

	Type of Impediment		
Degree	Consanguinity	Affinity	Illicit Affinity
1/1, 2/1, 1/2	7	22	47
2/2, 2/3, 3/2	96	13	63
3/3	69	7	*
3/4, 4/3, 4/4	47	3	*
TOTAL	219	45	110**
Percent of Marriages (N=2926)	7.5	1.5	5.6

*Not prohibited by canon law.
** Excluding twenty with multiple impediments and thirty-four of "hidden" or unknown degree.
Source: Petorca Parish, Marriage Registers.

are an accurate guide. Fully three out of four couples seeking the dispensation of consanguineous impediments cited sexual commerce as justification, and one-half had conceived at least one child (Table 3.5). For those with an illicit affinal impediment the proportion was even higher. This impediment was in itself an indication of both sexual passion and promiscuity with a close relative of the espoused. Sexual license, particularly by males, pervades the historical record. More than one macho man declared his prowess at bedding not only the sister of his espoused, but her mother as well. The unhappy mine foreman took the honor of his bride and also despoiled two of her first cousins. In 1837, the Archbishop dispensed an illicit affinal impediment for a Petorca couple "provided that the bride was born before the groom had intercourse with the mother." The priest had written of the "impediment of hidden affinity for illicit intercourse in the first degree '*linea recta*.' Also this bad amity lasted a long time; and the mother of the girl and the petitioner who wishes to marry the daughter are divorced from the sin and promise not to commit it again." The wide disparity in age between husband and wife facilitated extraordinarily rich combinations of unions and impediments. In the 1880s one groom aged twenty-six years had "illicit relations with the daughter of the bride's sister," while another aged thirty-five had "bad relations with . . . the sister of the bride and . . . the mother of the bride" who was twenty-seven and had children sired by the groom to legitimate. Multiple impediments--in an example from 1888,

TABLE 3.5
Justifications for dispensation of impediments to marriage: Petorca, 1840-1894

Justification	Impediment Type Consanguinity	Affinity	Illicit Affinity
Illicit commerce	38%	36%	48%
Progeny	28	23	39
Pregnant bride	9	5	22
Poverty	71	57	91
Lack of alternatives	51	30	31
Publicity	45	43	36
Advanced age of bride	22	25	25
Orphaned bride	24	20	18
Others	48	57	40
Total marriages (N)*	219	44	116
Total reasons cited (N)	736	149	360
Reasons/marriage	3.4	3.4	3.1

*Excluding those with reasons unspecified.
Source: Parish Marriage Records.

the groom's nephew had copulated with the bride, and the groom had done the same with her first cousin--were not absolute obstacles to marriage. A wedding in 1885 grew out of a sibling exchange: the groom admitted sexual intercourse with the bride's sister, the bride, with the groom's brother. In the end only one brother took a bride. Preference for sexual intercourse with several members within a single nuclear family was extraordinary. Fully one-third of grooms with affinal impediments admitted that they had copulated with the sister or mother of the betrothed. The corresponding proportion for brides was one of five. Whether this pattern reflects preference or spatial opportunities the statistical data cannot reveal. It does indicate significant premarital sexual promiscuity between families.

Dispensation records indicate that men were four times more likely to engage in illicit sex with a close relative of the ultimate bride, than women with kin of the future groom. Reasons for this disparity are unclear. Women who had already compromised their honor became less attractive as brides. In 35 percent of marriages with an illicit affinal impediment the difficulty of finding "another man because of the illicit commerce with the groom" or a similar phrase was cited as a justification for waiving the impediment. Women also had more reason to conceal their despoilment from the pretended and the priest. Nevertheless hidden impediments discovered after marriage usually indicate that the groom's honor was soiled rather than the bride's. A case from 1841 is typical. After two years of marriage a husband and wife

> . . . came to confession and they begged me . . . to absolve them of the affinity of first degree mixed with second in which X incurred (with his wife) for having had illicit copulation with the mother of his very wife before marriage and which the impediment was maliciously concealed when the nuptial testimony was taken so that her consent would not be annulled . . . .

Another husband, after twelve years of infertile marriage, attempted to use a deliberately concealed impediment in the first degree linea recta as an excuse to void the nuptial bonds. The vicar outmaneuvered him: "I have taken the measure of separating them after having had the delinquent imprisoned for publicizing his crime . . . . He has given proof of repentance and wishes to reform a new life." His wife died a few years later at age forty-six. The widower then took a seventeen-year old bride, who bore him a child within two years. Death struck again cutting short his enjoyment of paternal bliss and leaving a twenty-year old widow and an orphan.

The fragile position of women in the negotiation of a marriage is revealed by an instance of possible rape.

> After presenting the sworn nuptial testimonies . . . without describing any impediment for the celebration of the marriage an uncle by blood [of the groom] came forward assuring me that he had had sexual intercourse with [the bride]. I called her to me immediately, and only through great diligence could I obtain a confession from her of the act but denying that it had been voluntary on her part, rather that it had been the work of force carried out by the perpetrator. In the uncertainty that she might not be telling the truth, I threatened that I would not marry her if she did not confess the truth and finally she recanted, and has left me with the doubt of not knowing if she denied it from fear of losing the husband which was available to her or if she finally confessed because of the threat I made.

The Archbishop resolved the case by dispensing the impediment and having her say three Hail Marys. The lack of names in the affair prevents one from ascertaining whether she ultimately married. The ecclesiastical authorities seem to have ignored the uncle.

FINANCIAL IMPEDIMENTS TO MARRIAGE

If sexual license was so prevalent and women relatively powerless in the marriage market, why did Petorcans marry at all? The Church, parents, and social customs dictated that marriage was the conventional, desired form of conjugal union. Economic, social, psychological, and religious pressures ensured that a majority of adults married.

The Church's teachings and the vicars' exhortations strongly condemned sexual licentiousness and concubinage. Yet, the ultimate effect of Church policies was ambivalent. The parish priest urged his single parishioners to marry yet, at the same time, charged not insubstantial fees for the sacraments, erecting great obstacles to marriage for the poor. Records of parish visits by Archbishops and their secretaries reveal a long-standing concern over concubinage. Dr. D. Manuel Vicuña in his visit of 1838 instructed that

> . . . to avoid the concubinages which are enshrouded with the appearances of marriage and the demoralization of those who are truly married, the vicar will take special care to avoid the voluntary separation of spouses . . . and always when married strangers appear demand credentials which substantiate their marital status.

Vicars often conducted missions in the countryside to encourage peasants and their companions to sanctify their unions and end promiscuity. Not infrequently, a groom signed a statement promising "to reform his bad life abstaining absolutely from the excesses committed up to now." The logic of the Church's position must have seemed strange to the untutored poor. Consider the case of a literate groom of the prominent Olmos clan who wished to marry in 1875, but was prevented from doing so by an illicit affinity--carnal commerce with an aunt of the bride. Statements were taken and reported to the ecclesiastical authorities in the capital. Over a period of four months they responded with delays and requests for further testimony. The groom's initial justification was limited to "the public notoriety of the marriage and should it not occur . . . the grave prejudice for the bride." Following a request for further information, the groom replied that there were no additional justifications for the dispensation, but he would agree to increase his contribution to nine pesos. Still unsatisfied, the secretaries demanded more serious causes. The groom's response that the betrothed was pregnant failed to obtain succor. Finally the groom signed a statement that he had initially had sex with her "to abuse her and then abandon her," not to create a pretext for the dispensation. Only after she became pregnant did he change his mind. With this testimony the dispensation was promptly granted and the fee collected.

The ardor of parishioners to marry for "the tranquility of the soul" was tempered by the substantial charges for waiving formal requirements--impediments, the publication of marriage bans, and the three-week waiting period between the taking of testimony and the nuptial benediction--in addition to other less formal contributions. For three-quarters of a century civil authorities fought an intermittent political battle with the Church over the schedule of fees. In 1811, only one year after the struggle for independence erupted, the Junta de Gobierno ordered parish priests to provide the sacraments free of charge. The vicar of Petorca copied the order in the parish books (November 9, 1811), testily adding that the Junta would be held completely responsible for the consequences. Immediately upon the victory of the royal armies in 1814 the order was overturned and fees collected once again. A law promulgated in 1825 exempted the poorest day laborers, the gañanes, from marriage fees, but many neglected to take advantage of the privilege.[4] Relations between church and state constituted the most divisive political controversy of the nineteenth century. The issues were finally settled by the Civil Registry Act of 1884 which established a secular registration system and set a flat rate of fifty centavos for marriage sacraments and dispensations. Until 1885 marriage fees were negotiated between the vicar and the couple, taking into account impediments, special requests, and the petitioners' means.

The vicar, almost wholly dependent upon fees to maintain himself and the parish, experienced a conflict between his material wants and his parishioners' needs. In 1831 a wretched day laborer, whose wages were one real per day (12.5 centavos) paid six pesos and waited four months to obtain a dispensation for illicit affinity in the second degree. The vicar summed up the desperate situation as follows: "in addition to being a gañan he maintains a parcel of brothers and sisters recently orphaned of both parents who perished from smallpox." Vicars recognized the quandary of the poor, but invariably believed that the charity and mercy of the Church was underestimated. Consider this statement written in 1830:

> . . . for a long time [X and Y] lived in illicit friendship with such public scandal that they were denounced to me by the judges. Both showed the most ardent desire to extricate themselves from their unhappy state . . . , the reason being the utmost misery to which they had been reduced and their absolute lack of an offering to plead the dispensation which they need for their temporal and spiritual improvement. Oh, unfortunate ones! They have no idea of the fervent charity and paternal love of your Excellency's heart whose sole desire is the eternal salvation of the flock which has been entrusted to your care . . . .

Other vicars believed the marriage fee should be exploited

to encourage a higher morality in the poor. In 1853 a gañan who sought to take advantage of his exemption from fees would have been disappointed had he been able to read of the priest's efforts to dissuade the superiors from granting the dispensation:

> . . . in addition to having come together scandalously, trusting in the ease with which their impediments would be waived, this marriage has been made even more notorious by the protection of the patrones in whose house they work . . . . It should also be noted that in Chincolco concubinage between relatives is very frequent and it is feared that the news of its free dispensation will open the gates to such unions. The causes are diminished . . . by the woman having had children by other men, by her being completely capable of earning her own way and because the education of her children would not thereby be improved at all. Considering that she earns a salary for her work and he another, they can give at least twelve pesos.

The Archbishop granted the request without charge.

Approximately one-third of marriage inscriptions with impediments do not have a fee indicated. At least a portion probably paid something but the amount went unrecorded. For those who did pay, the fees were substantial, varying by the type and degree of impediment (Table 3.6). Charges for dispensing impediments of illicit affinity averaged five pesos, consanguinity, $7.30, and legal affinity, $7.67. These fees represented two or three months wages for poorer families and even an entire month's salary for a foreman, boss, or artisan. For poorer Petorcans nuptial fees were probably a greater restraint on formal marriage than parental consent or the lack of housing. Some parishioners went elsewhere to marry, thereby concealing the impediment and avoiding the necessarily greater fees. Occasionally "the patron of the petitioner obligated himself to pay the fine that you may impose," but often the gañan was left to his own means, which usually resulted in prolonged concubinage, a fact of which the priests were aware. In 1829, the vicar of Petorca resolved:

> Having taken notice in the missions in the countryside that some live publicly in illicit friendship I have decided to fulfill my duty by administering marriage to those who by their extreme poverty and ignorance of the exemption conceded to the day laborers have not come forward and thereby avoid scandal among the rest . . . . Displaying the extremely unhappy state in which they are found, they swore that as a result of impediments and their absolute poverty they remain for a long time without hope of remedy, confessing one groom that once he sought help but lacking the wherewithal to pay the dispensation he continued in the same life until the present.

TABLE 3.6
Fees for waiving marital impediments Petorca Parish, 1840-1884

Degree	Impediment Type								
	Consanguinity			Affinity			Illicit Affinity		
	$\overline{X}$	σ^2	N	$\overline{X}$	σ^2	N	$\overline{X}$	σ^2	N
1	$12.33	102.3	6	$5.40	7.1	5	$3.98	21.7	21
2	9.70	91.1	36	7.40	44.6	5	5.45	34.4	52
Other	6.07	43.1	94	8.95	41.4	10	--	--	--
Total	7.30	--	134	7.67	--	20	5.02	--	73
Fee not indicated*			46			18			34

*Excluding inscriptions with sparse information on most variables.
Source: Parish Records.

The enactment of the Civil Registry Laws freed the poor from onerous marriage duties but did not reduce concubinage. On the contrary the annulment of registration fees and a drastic reduction of parish charges were accompanied by a cheapening of the significance of marriage and a sharp decline in the marriage rate.[5] The law makers in the capital sought to alleviate the poor from an exorbitant expense and guarantee their offspring equitable, juridically sound succession to the patrimony. But for the poor people of Petorca marriage was mainly a religious duty and a spiritual, rather than legal, contract. Landless, but proud of their religious fervor, many did not immediately embrace the idea of civil marriage. For example, in 1885, a tenant farmer of modest means (behind two years in rental payments) paid fifty cents to the priest to obtain a dispensation of an impediment of legal affinity in the first degree to marry his deceased wife's sister. Citing poverty and public scandal, he sought to legitimate progeny born since his wife's death. The couple did not obtain a civil marriage until twenty-five years later, after procreating six children all of whom had been considered illegitimate under the law.

The civil authorities were not as inquisitive about sexual habits or conjugal preferences as long as incest with the immediate family and collateral consanguines to the second degree was avoided. Nor did the registrars exact excessive fees. For registrants who appeared during regular office hours, the civil authority was bound by law to inscribe the act and provide one notarized copy free of charge.[6] As the material benefits of civil marriage increased so did its acceptance by the general populace.

Parents also encouraged their children to marry. If prolonged celibacy was the status most preferred by parents for their children, early marriage was more desirable than concubinage. The documented instances of parents encouraging their children to wed rather than maintain public concubinage make up slightly less than 10 percent of marriages with impediments during the period 1840-1894. By law parental consent was required for persons marrying at less than twenty-five years of age. The 10 percent figure would seem to be instances where parents expressed their displeasure at their wayward children, invariably the daughter, by forcing them to marry rather than continue their sexual courting or concubinage. In 1850, seeking dispensation of a consanguineous impediment for a young pregnant woman, the vicar related that her father "cruelly punishes his daughter for her illicit dealings." Another woman, aged twenty-four, took refuge with the village authorities after her parents threw her into the street. Adopted children sometimes suffered a similar fate: "some time ago because of the hope of marriage, the girl had lost her place in the house where she had been brought up." In 1845 a sixteen-year old girl wished to marry a miner aged twenty, but was obstructed by his having had intercourse with her aunt. Upon learning of the pregnancy, the parents punished her, "driving her out of her mind." Another girl, aged twenty-four, impeded by a consanguineous tie (3/3) sought to marry a recently widowed teamster; meanwhile the bride's parents heaped heavy work and abuse on her because of the dishonor she had experienced by him. Sons enjoyed a less demanding standard of conduct. There are no examples of a father reprimanding a son for sexual promiscuity. The ultimate effect of parental authority was ambiguous. On the one side, many parents sought to delay the marriage of their children and influence the choice of spouse; on the other hand, delay increased the risk that sexual passion would overcome the power of parental restraints and end with the loss of virginity and family honor.

LEGACIES FOR NATURAL CHILDREN

Parental pressures and the moral authority of the Church combined with social prejudice against illegitimacy and concubinage to encourage young people to form stable unions and marry. If sexual promiscuity by males was acceptable, even encouraged, it was deplored for women, particularly those of the better class. Less than 10 percent of testatrices admitted bearing natural children before marriage. This figure includes one will (of 193 by married women) in which natural children were recognized. The figure should have been two or three times as great if the norm estimated from genealogical histories is accurate. The proportion for single women was three times greater,

TABLE 3.7
Frequency of natural children in wills by sex and marital status of testator, 1825-1970

	Men		Women	
Natural Children	Married	Single	Married	Single
No	191	18	176	64
Yes	32	10	17	18

Source: NP.

but this level is somewhat lower than one would expect from the general level of illegitimacy (Table 3.7 and Figure 3.1). Once again the more relaxed moral code for males is evident here. Male testators were 1.4 times more likely to mention natural children as females. Nevertheless, for women, the degree of misfortune arising from sexual promiscuity or concubinage could be reduced by choosing a partner of equal or higher social rank. One wealthy lady proudly related in her will that while she had remained a life-long spinster, she "had [three surviving] natural children sired by a person of quality corresponding to my birth, good name and reputation."[7]

For Petorcans with something to bestow upon their heirs concubinage was even less frequently recognized than outright illegitimacy. Among the surviving wills, there is a single instance of someone recognizing five or more natural children with the same partner. In this case, dated 1949, the testator was certainly not a member of the elite. A poor bachelor tenant farmer bequeathed to his five natural children five cows, four calves, two yearlings, one horse, a filly, and a donkey in addition to a tiny sum of cash.[8] Among the truly better-off, extramarital sex seems to have been a trifling affair. The listings of natural children show considerable sexual mobility for both men and women. Of thirty-four wills with more than one natural child, only six indicate more than one child by the same person. The cases related above are the only ones which could be considered concubinages. Of seventy-five testators with natural children, only eighteen indicated more than two.

Both concubinage and illegitimacy were much more common among the poor, who because of their wretchedness and misery could afford little else. The relationship between illegitimacy and poverty accentuated the offensiveness of both. Not infrequently an accommodated bastard sought to conceal illegitimate origins. In 1843 a young groom wishing to marry into one of the valley's wealthier families requested the vicar to not announce the bans from the altar on three successive Sundays "because of the shame it would cause me to make my illegitimacy so public." Although delayed for four years (the reasons for the prolonged delay are not indicated), the wedding eventually occurred and without the publication of bans. Frequently the Church received an offering of ten pesos and even more for this type of dispensation, a privilege reserved for the wealthy who, to save face, could afford to spend the equivalent of a gañan's wages for a half year. The embarrassment caused by illegitimate origins were shared by all classes. In 1870 a twenty-four year old woman of natural origins suffered the humiliation of being refused even implicit recognition by her biological, but unmarried parents. Each had since married someone else and refused to receive any communication from her. After three months of depositions and petitions, a guardian was appointed by the Courts to provide the juridically required consent. The groom was twenty years older than she, and also illegitimate and illiterate.

In the parish records the word "concubinage" is frequently associated with "desgraciado" (miserable, unfortunate, disgraceful). The pertinacity that Petorcans might display to escape from what they considered a disgraceful state is illustrated by the case of a poor teamster in 1852. The priest observed:

> . . . only because of the great desire to marry his cousin could have made him offer three ounces of gold, equivalent to forty or more ounces for a rich man, thus it is that although his reasons are not very strong, I fear that the desire of this man would maintain him in his bad life and I consider it a great sacrifice to put up this amount and nevertheless he offers it. In this was I think everything to have been reconciled.

Illegitimacy not only inflicted opprobrium on the offspring, life chances were reduced as well. Most bastards were supported solely by their mothers or the maternal family, if by any biological kin at all. Abandonment was not uncommon. Few bastards obtained support or even recognition from their fathers. The notice given natural children in wills was more often limited to a grudging acknowledgement to forestall further claims or to document what the father believed to have been a generous prior settlement in supporting the offspring's maintenance. In a will dated 1885 a married man from a respected family simply dismissed the fruits of a wayward life as "two natural children whose names and domicile I don't recall."[9] Others used testaments to limit the inheritance of the natural child. A married testatrix, lacking legitimate offspring, declared her husband as her sole heir and then noted: "before marrying a natural child, Carmelita . . . , was born to me which exists yet in Chincolco and I give her twenty pesos, a kerchief, one silk dress and two small gold chains, with this separating her from any right to my goods."[10] A bachelor began the clause dealing with his natural children thusly: ". . . no greater rights should be given [my two natural children] than those set down in this testament . . . ."[11] This testator, lacking direct legitimate heirs, left most of his possessions to a cousin, alloting to the bastard daughter, "should she reach majority," a small plot ("poseciончita") "by which I completely divorce her from my goods," and to the son, "should he attain majority," a saddled horse. Future, conditional, and subjunctive tenses are more common in statements of bequeathals to bastards. Slim life chances, restricted rights before the law, and the parent's resistance to spreading a meager inheritance--all of these factors encouraged testators to change moods in stating their legacies for their natural children.

Other parents demonstrate considerable affection and equity for their illegitimate heirs, but such was not the norm. In 1872 one aged woman singled out two illegitimate grandchildren orphaned through the death of her own children to ensure that they received their due.[12] When one of these more fortunate children was baptized, the grandparents actually appeared as parents in the baptismal record! There is only one instance of a testator explicitly declaring heirs "in equal parts, my children, legitimate and natural."[13] This involved a widowed woman of limited means with only one legitimate child.

THE MESTIZO MARRIAGE PATTERN

Sexual passion, the moral authority of the Church, community mores, and parental power combined to encourage a majority of Petorcans, both male and female, to marry. The average age at marriage was remarkably similar to those in Western Europe before the industrial revolution (Table 3.8).[14] For almost 5,000 first marriages celebrated in Petorca over the past 130 years, the mean age for women was 25.3 years, exactly identical to the average for forty European communities over the period 1600-1849 as computed from family history studies. Petorca men married on average only 2.5 months later than European men. However, the beginnings of family life in Petorca differed greatly from that of European peasant communities of the past such as Colyton (Devon) and Crulai (Normandy).[15] Prenuptial sexual courtship, concubinage, and illicit copulation--integral states in the lives of most adult, even adolescent, Petorcans--were almost unknown in Colyton and Crulai. In the Petorca Valley, family life began more naturally, without the intrusion of law, whether of the church or the state. The transitions from courtship and coupling to

TABLE 3.8
Family beginnings in Petorca and the average age at marriage in historical Western Europe

	Bride	Groom
Mean age at first marriage (years)		
Western Europe, 1600-1849	25.3	27.8
Petorca, 1840-1969	25.3	28.0
N	4920	4175
Mean age at coupling (years)		
Petorca, 1840-1969	22.7	--
N	5211	--

NOTE: Figures for Western Europe are the unweighted average for forty villages as reported by Gaskin.

Source: Gaskin, "Age at First Marriage," p. 29. Marriages Dataset.

conjugality followed a more individual rhythm, impelled or retarded by the subtle interplay of personal preferences and physiological fecundity. The intermixing of three biocultures--Indian, European, and, to a much lesser extent, African--within a dualistic economy of dependence and subsistence produced a mestizo marriage pattern, characterized by early age at coupling and considerable pre- and extramarital fertility. Adjustments for the beginning of fertile sexual activity indicate that for Petorcans the average age of pairing was more nearly 22.7 years, about two and one-half years before marriage.

The demographic and social implications of the age difference between juridical and natural union were considerable. Lengthening the fertility cycle of women during their most fecund years and shortening the span of generations substantially increased the rate of population growth. The richer possibilities of more complex family structures, greater interaction across generations and the slower tempo of economic opportunities arising from generational succession--all derive from the younger ages of natural, as opposed to juridical, family beginnings.[16] For Petorcans, then, marriage age was of less significance than the age of coupling or pairing, the moment or process of coming together ultimately leading to marriage. The age of coupling may be estimated by taking into account ages at marriage and the births of first children, both legitimate and natural. While there is only sporadic confirmation that any particular prenuptial conception may be the fruit of intercourse between a specified bride and her legal mate, for practical purposes the complications of establishing paternity may be laid aside.[17] Although the consensual nature of pairings prevented their being recorded, information about marriage and prenuptial birth or conception dates can be used to estimate an age of coupling for each connubial family. For unions beginning with marriage (Type "M", i.e. no attributable prenuptial conceptions), the date of coupling is simply defined as the date of marriage. For other types of marriages, the date of the bride's first parturition and the interval between marriage and birth for Type M unions is used to estimate the date of union. For 1296 Type M marriages with at least one legitimate birth, the average protogenesique interval was 1.8 years or 21.6 months. For brides with prenuptial births, Type "B" unions, subtracting 1.8 years from the age of the first prenuptial birth attributed to each bride--21.3 years for the period 1840-1862--yields the female age of pairing (the mean for this period is 21.3 - 1.8 = 19.5; see Table 3.9). Similarly, for brides actually pregnant at marriage and no record of prenuptial birth (Type "C"), the age of coupling is derived by subtracting the average Type M protogenesique interval (21.6 months) less the average number of months pregnant at marriage for Type C brides (3.6 months) from the corresponding age of marriage (for the first period the average is 22.3 - 1.5 = 20.8).[18] The resulting variable, the age at which unions occurred ultimately leading to matrimony irrespective of type, provides a more parsimonious indicator of the beginning of family life without the complications of controlling for type of union, the age at which prenuptial births occurred, and the like.

The distribution of specific types of family unions varied from 5 to 15 percent from one period to another. While marriage was always the dominant mode of initiating unions, ranging from 43 to 50 percent of all types, consensual unions which led to marriage were almost as common (36-43 percent). The proportion of brides pregnant at marriage with no prenuptial births varied within the narrow range of 12.7 to 14.4 percent. These figures, representing the experience of all brides marrying in the community, are biased to a certain extent by the effects of geographical mobility. Women who moved before or shortly after marrying were less likely to have registered a prenuptial birth in the study area. Selecting a geographically stable subset of marital unions reduces the percentage of Type M brides and increases proportionally other types (Table 3.11). These data provide additional convincing arguments for using an unconventional date for the beginning of unions. Finally the association between marriage type and measured social variables--literacy, occupation, legitimacy and migration--further illustrates the need for a more realistic indicator of the beginning of unions. The relationship between social status and marriage type is not surprising. Groups of higher status were more apt to begin family life with marriage than others. Over 65 percent of merchants, bureaucrats, teachers,

TABLE 3.9
Age at coupling estimated from ages at marriage and first legitimate birth: Petorca, 1840-1969

	Marriage Period				
	1840-1862	1863-1894	1895-1929	1930-1969	Unweighted Average
First Marriages of Women with One Legitimate Birth and No History of Prenuptial Conceptions					
Mean age (years)					
First Birth (a)	23.50	24.69	25.40	22.52	24.05
Marriage (b)	21.62	23.07	23.48	20.85	22.25
Protogenesique interval (a-b)	1.88	1.72	1.92	1.67	1.80
N	287	396	228	385	324
First Marriage of Women with One or More Prenuptial Births					
First legitimate birth*	25.92	28.26	28.41	26.20	27.20
Marriage	24.99	27.64	28.10	27.09	26.95
First prenuptial birth (c)	21.32	22.70	23.02	21.39	22.11
Coupling (c-1.8)	19.56	20.90	21.22	19.61	20.85
N	453	545	459	596	513

* Not directly comparable to subsequent variables which include unions with no legitimate birth within study area.

Dataset: Marriages.

TABLE 3.10
Distribution and average age at marriage by type of family beginning (first marriage for bride)

	Marriage Period			
	1840-1862	1863-1894	1895-1929	1930-1969
Relative distribution				
Marriage	46.3%	49.6%	42.7%	47.8%
Prenuptial conception	13.9	14.0	14.4	12.7
Prenuptial birth	39.8	36.3	43.0	39.5
N	1051	1398	1001	1413
Average age at marriage				
All types	23.8	25.9	26.6	24.5
Marriage	23.2	25.1	26.0	23.2
Prenuptial conception	22.3	23.9	24.2	21.3
Prenuptial birth	25.0	27.6	28.1	27.1
Average age at first prenuptial birth	21.3	22.7	23.0	21.4
Average age at coupling	21.8	23.7	23.8	21.7

Dataset: Marriages.

TABLE 3.11
Marriages by type of family beginning and period for selected unions

	Marriage Period			
	1840-1862	1863-1894	1895-1929	1930-1969
Type of beginning				
Marriage (M)	44.3%	45.9%	34.3%	41.5%
Prenuptial birth (B)	40.3	37.3	47.7	41.9
Prenuptial conception (C)	15.4	16.8	18.0	16.5
N	591	603	239	508
"B" and bride pregnant at marriage (B^1)	8.5	8.6	13.4	13.2
Total brides pregnant ($C+B^1$)	23.9	25.4	31.4	29.7
No. of natural children (type "B" marriages)				
One	58.8	57.3	44.7	47.9
Two	22.7	24.4	22.8	22.5
Three	11.8	9.8	6.1	10.3
Four or more	6.7	8.4	26.3	19.3
N	238	225	114	213

Dataset: Select Marriages.

and the like initiated unions with marriage while miners and farmers did so much less often (47 and 43 percent, respectively). For marriages in which both bride and groom are literate, 57 percent had no record of prenuptial conceptions. At the opposite end of the literacy scale, with both spouses illiterate, only 43 percent began with marriage. For legitimate brides and grooms, the figure was 50 percent and for others 43 percent. The age at coupling, then, facilitates comparative analysis of the beginning of family life without the need for specifying family type.

PERIODIZATION OF MARRIAGE COHORTS

A brief discussion of periodization is necessary before proceeding. Four broad periods--1840-1862, 1863-1894, 1895-1929, and 1930-1969--were selected to summarize major change in the patterns of family beginnings and fertility in the valley. Although the undercurrents of population history flow slowly, shifting direction on a scale of decades rather than years, arbitrary annual cutting points have been selected to simplify the discussion. Each date marks a turning point in the population history of the valley. Eighteen forty is the earliest year for which sufficiently reliable data exist to permit the construction of family genealogies.[19] From the wars of independence to the late 1830s parish records were kept chaotically and the sacraments were administered sporadically, if at all (see Appendix I). The second turning point began in the 1860s when the population density of the valley peaked, epidemics struck with increasing frequency and severity, and population pressure encouraged growing numbers of Petorcans to migrate. Eighteen ninety-five marks more of a turning point in population record keeping than any real change in demographic levels. Given the traditional skepticism about the relative efficiency of the civil compared with the parochial registration system, it is essential to differentiate between the two eras. Finally, 1930 signals the beginning of the greatest population changes to occur in the valley since its settlement in the eighteenth century: dramatic declines in the age at marriage, in death rates, and eventually in birth rates as well.

The overall age of first marriage for women rose from 23.8 years for the period 1840-1862 to a plateau of 26 years and persisted at that level for two-thirds of a century.[20] In the 1930s a substantial decline set in. Movements in marriage age by union type parallel the general average. Period effects are much more important in determining nuptial age than shifts between types of beginnings. Nevertheless, the conventional indicator poorly estimates the age of union for women with prenuptial births. For this group the average age of marriage confounds the timing of pairings with the relative attractiveness of the legal formalities of marriage. During the period 1863-1894 the increasing popularity of legal unions is demonstrated by a very large rise in average marriage age for brides with prenuptial births (2.6 years), while the average age at first prenuptial birth only increased by about half as much. Similarly period effects for Type B unions from 1895 to 1969 are much greater than that indicated by the evolution in marriage age. The average age of marriage for Type B brides declines by 3.5 percent from 28.1 to 27.1 years; however, the average at first prenuptial birth declines by 7.0 percent from 23.0 to 21.4 years.

Comparing the differences between the level and degree of change in the coupling statistic with the conventional marriage indicator reveals the shortcomings of the latter wherever prenuptial births are common. The average age at coupling shows a much simpler pattern in the timing of unions in Petorca. Over the 130 year period there were only two levels of average age at first unions, each separated by two years. For the first and last period the average was 21.8 years rising to 23.8 for the period 1863-1929. Until 1895 the indicators move in lock step, separated by exactly two years. For the period 1895-1929, the conventional measure suggests a delay in marriage, not apparent in the mean age for forming unions. For the latest period the margin of difference is greater yet. The mean age of coupling shows that in recent years the women of Petorca were apparently beginning family life slightly earlier than during any period in the past.

PRECOCIOUS COUPLINGS, 1840-1862

For women marrying during the period 1840-1862, the age at pairing off must be characterized as precocious. The mean age at coupling was slightly less than twenty-two years, more than three years below the average age of marriage for the Western European standard. If women with no record of legitimate offspring (including both sterile women and those who migrated after marriage) are deleted the figure falls by an additional year to 20.9. Both age at pairing and marriage is strongly associated with relative fecundity. Nonmigrating, fertile women married two years earlier than others (23.0 vs. 24.9) and started families four years sooner. The first legitimate birth for the typical couple occurred over four years after the beginning of a pairing which had already produced two children. This mestizo pattern of family formation encouraged both precocious family beginnings and apparently made for more fertile matches than might have taken place if prenuptial intercourse had not been the custom. Total legitimate fertility rates for Type B and C unions averaged some 15 percent greater than those for Type M women. Moreover, the differential becomes even greater if only older marrying women are considered. Comparing cumulative legitimate fertility at ages 30-44, we find that for women marrying in their teens the fertility differential is insignificant, less than 10 percent. It rises slightly to 14 percent for women marrying at ages 20-24, but peaks for late marrying women (ages 25-29) at over 50 percent (see Table 4.10). Most Petorcan women, then, had borne two births before the age at which women of Colyton or Crulai had even married; moreover, they seemed to continue with relatively higher birth rates than would otherwise have been possible if courting customs had not maximized the fecundity of individual couples. These factors in combination provide a partial explanation for the much higher rates of population increase found in Latin America in earlier centuries. Where European populations grew at perhaps 0.5 percent per year over long periods, the Chilean population increased at 1.0-1.5 percent throughout much of the nineteenth century. More reliable mortality estimates than those available for Petorca and studies of other communities are needed to construct a convincing proof.[21]

DEMOGRAPHIC CRISIS AND THE DELAY OF COUPLING, 1863-1894

Beginning in the 1850s, increasing population density fostered by the growth momentum of earlier years, worsening economic conditions, and drought produced a subsistence crisis followed by a prolonged period of hard times. The demographic response was twofold: marriage restraint--the preventive check, the delaying of marriage, or its avoidance altogether--and migration. These transformations of the demographic rhythms persisted for several generations, through the 1920s.

Epidemics were not uncommon in Petorca, but those of the 1860s and 1870s were probably more severe than any in the valley's history. Accompanied by prolonged drought, partially the result of deforestation from mining and overgrazing of livestock, Petorcans were hard-pressed to maintain their livelihood. Farming was always somewhat marginal in the valley, but the absence of rains in 1863 and beyond led to a great dearth of grains and other foods. In 1864 an exceptionally persistent, very deadly typhoid epidemic devastated the community. According to the governor's report for that year:

> . . . an infinite multitude has perished before one's eyes for a lack of resources to combat the havoc of the mortiferous epidemic of typhoid fever that has snatched away so many lives in this department [county], which has no druggist, blood-letter, mid-wife or even a simple lover of medicine; on the contrary, the unfortunate sick must fall into the hands of stupid quacks who live in the countryside and concoct their remedies like witches . . . .
>
> In the meantime we went naked, experienced famine and saw sick ones perish without being able to succor them in

> any way whatsoever . . . .[22]

Within two years the great drought intensified, causing further scarcity and hardship. The grotesque character of an economy trapped between subsistence and dependence is illustrated in a letter of 1867:

> The drought during the winter powerfully affected the grain harvest, making it much less abundant than in the past; and as a little later the great export of wheat [to Britain] took place, there flocked from everywhere merchants in search of this article and the holders, faced with a price unknown until now, did not take into account that they should reserve seeds necessary for sowing as well as that for food. Naturally, soon there developed an extreme shortage in the department which reached such an extreme that many people did not dare to sow fearing that afterwards they would lack that necessary for the sustenance of their families.[23]

Shortly a public seed granary was established to ensure sowing reserves for the poor. Nevertheless, the crisis persisted. In 1872, 1874, and 1878, typhoid, "membrana," and smallpox epidemics followed in rapid succession.[24]

The demographic effects of hardship are reflected in even the crude population figures. In the 1860s baptisms stabilized and began a long secular decline at the same time that the number of burials soared to unsurpassed heights and remained at a rather high plateau into the 1880s (Figure 2.4). The family histories permit a more refined assessment of the effects of ecological and economic decay. Both the mean age at marriage and coupling rose by some two years to 25.9 and 23.7, respectively (Table 3.12). The delay in age at pairing was greatest for brides of farmers (2.4 years) and least for those of grooms with urbane occupations (1.6 years). At the same time the proportion of brides aged less than twenty-five years declined by almost one-quarter. Not only did Petorca men and women delay marriage, a much greater proportion remained celibate until death. Moreover, the effects of sexual courting customs were transformed such that more fecund women seem to have become less attractive as potential mates. In any case, during a period of rising illegitimacy, fewer brides had prenuptial births. Older women with relatively more natural children were much less likely to marry than in previous years. Changes in fertility levels during this period cannot be ascertained with precision because of the high error rate (10 to 30 percent for pre-1860 cohorts). Moreover, following the conventions of historical demography, fertility data were tabulated by birth and marriage cohorts rather than by periods. Accepting the data with a certain degree of error in omissions and periodization, we find that for the cohort of women born 1820-1840 and bearing children from 1840-1885,

TABLE 3.12
The preventive check: demographic responses to population pressure

	Marriage Period		
	1840-1862	1863-1895	Percentage Difference
Female mean age at first coupling	21.8	23.7	9
Female mean age at first marriage	23.8	25.9	9
Male mean age at first marriage	27.1	28.5	5
Brides aged 12-24 (percent of all brides)	58.6	45.8	-22
Female permanent celibacy (%)	20.5	29.8	45
Brides 30+ with 2+ prenuptial children (%)*	39.2	27.6	-30
Illegitimacy (percent of total births)	20.0	26.9	35

Datasets: Marriages, *Select Marriages, Adult Deaths, Linkable Births.

NOTE: Permanent celibacy is calculated from deaths of women aged 45-64 dying in study area and born 1800-1834 and 1835-1869, respectively. Births refer to 1840-1864 and 1865-1894 regardless of mother's birthplace.

total legitimate fertility was 15 percent less than for the immediately preceding cohort which bore children from 1820-1865. Moreover, the decline was largest and most persistent for Type M wives. Their rates dropped by one-fifth and did not regain the higher level until 1900 and beyond. For wives of other types of unions the decline was only 12 percent and recovered with the following cohort.[25] The significance of the demographic crisis of this period is not that it was particularly horrifying on any absolute scale; rather, that faced with a deterioration in living conditions, Petorcans responded with personal decisions which alleviated at least to a small degree the demographic pressures which were to a certain extent responsible for their misery.

ADMINISTRATIVE CHANGE AND STABLE COUPLING PATTERNS, 1895-1929

Changes in family formation patterns from 1895 to 1929 were more administrative than real. The relatively later age of pairing established during the decades of adversity persisted into the twentieth century, undisturbed by the transition from registering sacraments to vital events. The mean age of marriage increased by almost one year, but the age of coupling remained constant. The movement in the former was produced by a redistribution of the manner by which families were begun. Only one in three brides began family life with marriage while almost half bore at least one child before registering their union with the state. The proportion of Type M marriages declined by 25 percent with a corresponding increase in Type B weddings. The largest relative changes occurred in the proportion of brides with four or more prenuptial births--up two-fold--while those with one child before marriage declined by one-fourth. Almost one out of three brides was pregnant at marriage. The effect of these developments on the timing of unions was virtually nil. If women and particularly men married at older ages than ever, they were not delaying the transition from celibacy to coupling but rather from coupling to marriage. Men on average married at thirty years of age, but seem likely to have entered consensual unions several years sooner.

Three substantively important changes in family beginnings did occur during this period. The mean age of coupling for subsequently fecund brides began a decline--very likely the result of rising fecundity at younger ages--which would accelerate greatly after 1930. During this period, the differentiation in family formation patterns by occupational groups became inverted. In both earlier and later periods middle class brides, because of their disposition for initiating families with marriage, coupled some two years later than other groups. However, during the years 1895-1929, this differential temporarily disappeared. The average age at female pairing for all occupational groups (except miners) ranged between 23.1 and 23.8 years, with middle-class brides at the mid-point. Miners responded to the depressed state of their industry by delaying pairing to the relatively old age of twenty-five years for women. The mean delay in marriage for men was only about six months to thirty-one years. The total population of the valley declined considerably during this period and legal marriage became a much less popular condition, but Petorcans did not in general further delay the timing of pairing.

THE NUPTIALITY TRANSITION, 1930-1970

Beginning in the 1930s a revolution occurred in family formation patterns. For females, both the average age at marriage and coupling fell sharply, some two years on average, accompanied by a substantial increase in the proportion of brides who began conjugal life with marriage (Table 3.13). As a result of younger average age at

TABLE 3.13
Marriage transition after the Great Depression

	Marriage Period		
	1895-1929	1930-1969	Percentage Difference
Female mean age at first coupling	23.8	21.7	-9
Female mean age at first marriage	26.1	24.0	-8
Male mean age at first marriage	30.0	28.4	-5
Brides aged 12-24 (percent of all brides)	49.8	70.1	41
Brides beginning family with marriage (%)*	38.7	47.2	22
Female permanent celibacy (%)	33.7	20.0	-41
Illegitimate births (%)	34.0	19.0	-44

Datasets: Marriage, *Select Marriages, Linkable Births.

NOTE: Permanent celibacy is calculated from deaths of women aged 45-64 dying in study area and born 1870-1904 and 1905-1919, respectively. Births refer to 1895-1929 and 1930-1969, regardless of mother's birthplace.

marriage the premarital pregnancy phase of courtship was avoided for about 20 percent more brides than in the previous period. The proportion of Type B brides declined, although their absolute numbers remained substantial. Almost 60 percent of unions legitimated by marriage included at least one premarital pregnancy. The increase in Type M brides was essentially a function of the changing age pattern of marriage. With relatively younger brides, the overall proportion of those having a premarital pregnancy declined although the proportion within specific age groups remained unchanged. Older spinsters with children also found their way to official marriage in much greater proportions than in other epochs. Aged single mothers, who in an earlier day would have remained concubines or abandoned mates, suddenly found the social or economic wherewithal to legitimize their conjugal arrangements. The restriction of government allowances to legitimate children was responsible for this to some extent, but rising living standards and expectations of a better life were probably important as well. Women, both young and old, who in earlier epochs would have delayed legal marriage for years, if not permanently, and meanwhile experienced several interruptions as partners drifted in and out, now settled quickly into institutionalized, legally sanctioned family life.

The most significant development was the declining age of coupling, which dropped well below twenty-two years. For some groups, such as brides of day laborers, the average age at pairing was less than twenty. Middle-class brides continued to initiate families between twenty-three and twenty-four, while brides marrying into other occupational groups paired off between twenty-one and twenty-two on the average. The effects of other social variables on mean age at coupling were slight. However, the age of coupling was highly correlated with fecundity. The increased fecundity of young women interacted with marriage mores to encourage very young ages of coupling and marriage. The average pairing age for brides who subsequently bore a child in the study area declined from 22.2 to 20.2 years, permitting a generational turnover of five times per century compared to less than four for European peasant communities of the past. Moreover, for the demonstrably most fecund group, brides who actually bore children before marriage, the average age was only 19.5 years compared to 20.0 for Type C brides and 23.9 for those who first married. While the effects of the increasing precocity of pairing is difficult to estimate precisely, accelerating population growth rates is obviously one important consequence.

The marriage revolution affected not only the timing of unions but also the degree of permanent celibacy. The proportion of females who never married dropped to a historic low. Juridically sanctioned marriage became the customary way of maintaining family life. The relative frequency of permanently natural children also fell to the lowest level ever in the valley. Nevertheless, the proportion of natural children remained high, about 20 percent of all births.

These innovations were made possible by the vast expansion of government services in the community and the development of attractive job opportunities both within and outside the valley, relieving residents of the responsibility for generating economic infrastructure at the same pace as the rate of biological reproduction. A small army of public bureaucrats, provided for by national tax revenues which the local economy often could not generate, gradually grew up in the valley. Hospital services incremented slowly but steadily and with them the staff increased from a half dozen paid employees when it first opened in 1885 to several score in recent years. Universal education required the founding of additional schools and eventually a vastly expanded teaching staff paid by the central government. Police, juridical, administrative, and social services expanded, providing additional sources of income for the local economy and insuring a certain economic vitality for the community. Programs to assist the small miners helped expand and then maintain production at several old mining operations. Government mining policies and price floors for the mines virtually guaranteed their continued operation and thereby jobs for as many as a hundred miners. Agricultural development programs, part of a broad national agrarian policy, were extended to the valley providing local farmers capital, seeds, knowledge, and modern technology to sustain the agricultural base for a larger portion of the community. While government policies at the national level were ambivalent--its pricing policies inhibited agricultural investment and encouraged low renumeration of farm labor--they probably prevented the complete demise of market farming for the marginal operations in the arid Norte Chico.

The explanation of innovations in family formation patterns is found in the structural transformation of the social, economic, demographic, and political conditions within the valley which in turn encouraged an increasingly wider circle of the populace to achieve the behavioral norms of more prosperous and socially powerful families. Family initiation patterns predominant in recent decades were anticipated by an elite of educated, prosperous couples more than a century ago. The transition was more than simply a matter of the gradual decay of a bastardy subculture, or the accretion of families who from generation to generation legitimated their unions. The process was one of acquiring both a stable livelihood and confident expectations for undertaking the additional responsibilities of marriage. The process was integral. Much of the impetus and the means came from outside. Nevertheless, as technical, economic, and social innovations--often unearned in the sense that the community did not develop them and often, in a commercial sense, could not pay for them--penetrated hamlet and farm, they wrought not only a social transformation, but a demographic one as well. Perhaps, at the outset, the demographic transition was essentially a mortality transition (see Chapter 5). Very quickly there followed a marriage transition as well, achieved by means of the same social, economic, administrative, and technological innovations which produced mortality changes: expanded education, improved communication and transportation, an efficacious public bureaucracy, and a diversified, perhaps more stable, local and national economy. Shortly this change was translated, if not into a higher standard of living, at least into the confidence that generally life was improving.

The principal determinants of family initiation patterns ending with marriage have always been economic and remain so today. As far as legitimate marriage is concerned, there does not seem to have ever existed anything approaching a caste of the illegitimate. Similarly, legitimate offspring have not invariably mimicked the marriage patterns of their parents. For generations, the proportions of illegitimates who married approximated their relative frequency at birth. Moreover, the rate of endogamy according to legitimacy of spouses has always been very low; marital partners seem to have been selected almost by chance as far as legitimacy is concerned. Finally, legitimate spouses were only slightly less likely than illegitimates to start a family with a natural child. The principal difference may have been that illegitimates simply did not enter the marriage stream according to their numbers in the larger population. Mortality and migration differentials by legitimacy status have probably been too great to accept, as conclusive proof, the quantitative correlation between cohort bastardy ratios and the frequency of illegitimacy at marriage.

If a bastardy subculture has not been important in the past, it seems likely to become so in the future. For many decades the community has been undergoing a process of differentiation in which homogeneous social, occupational, and economic structures have become increasingly heterogeneous. In the not too distant past, the principal educational differences were simple ones of literacy with illiterates making up some 80 percent of the population or more. For the most recent generation the figures have inverted, but within the broad mass very considerable differences exist--from university graduates to marginally functional literates. These gradations existed a century ago, but very few Petorcans counted themselves among the literate. Occupational differentiation developed along the same lines. While the valley does not yet have a numerically large middle class, there are widening differences between adults, families, and geographically specific areas of the valley. Village life has collapsed, but the villages remain.

Petorcans, integrated into a regional economy from the first settling, experienced the social ramifications of an expanding, dynamic, and diversified economy from the first stages of the process. Notwithstanding the economic stagnation of the local economy, the occupational structure of the valley became more complex in time with national developments. Class differentials became correspondingly more heterogeneous. The elite--the Portales, the Sepulveda, and the Montt families--saw an ever-growing middle group--the Lillos, the Gonzales, and others competing for a second rank niche in which a family might grow and prosper. Now with widening social and economic differentials, bastardy is confined increasingly to a homogeneous subgroup--the uneducated, illiterate, and illegitimate common laborers.

Nevertheless, considerable diversity of family formation patterns exists. These trends do not signify a return to the suffocating social immobility of the mid-nineteenth century. The extension of modern marriage patterns has not obliterated the importance of premarital pregnancy in encouraging people to marry. Petorcan courtship customs continue to favor the fertile.

Petorcans, today as in the past, are demographically sensitive to their social and economic circumstances, and this is reflected in both family formation patterns and, as will be shown, fertility levels. Whether they have a demographic calculus is not at issue. The facts are that Petorcans' marital patterns have shown pronounced flexibility in the face of changing economic and social circumstances. Their demographic responsiveness was so highly developed that during the crisis of the 1860s Petorcans seem to have selected less fecund women as brides more often than for earlier generations. Certainly, fewer brides had natural children and brides with natural children went to the altar less often than in other epochs. Recently, Petorcans' marital flexibility has been demonstrated anew with the very rapid acquisition of modern marriage patterns in the lifetime of a single generation.

NOTES

1. Peter Laslett (Family Life and Illicit Love in Earlier Generations [London, 1977], p. 108) notes that the English also referred to bastards as "natural" children.

2. Citations from marriage dispensation records are abbreviated to the year given in the text.

3. Ricardo Cruz-Coke ("A Genetic Reform of the Civil Law Computations of the Degrees of Relationship in Families," Social Biology, Vol. 24 [1978], pp. 93-99) compares civil computations with a genetic system, and discusses the various types of consanguinity. For a historical account of the evolution of the concept in Europe, see Jean-Louis Flandrin, Families in Former Times, Kinship, Household and Sexuality (London, 1979), pp. 19-33.

4. In the marriage book for 1825, the vicar wrote:

> As a result of the decree which absolves the gañanes of the fees for marriage and not having an endowed notary to maintain this archive with the formalities of process in its marriage testimonies, I have resolved, tired of doing this task free of charge, to only take their depositions to know if they do or do not have impediments, and keep only a brief account of what they declare and obtain their consent to procede to the bans and marry them.

5. Miguel Yrarrázaval Vera, Manual del rejistro civil para conocimiento de todos y especialmente de los oficiales del registro civil (Valparaiso, 1885), pp. 27-29. Crude marriage rates for Chile from 1850 to 1973 are reported in R. McCaa, "Chilean Social and Demographic History: Sources, Issues, and Methods," Latin American Research Review, Vol. 13 (1978), p. 114.

6. Yrarrázaval, Manual del rejistro civil, p. 51.

7. NP, Vol. 6, f. 407.

8. NP, Vol. 1949, f. 172.

9. NP, Vol. 1885, f. 98.

10. NP, Vol. 27, f. 58

11. NP, Vol. 46, f. 43.

12. NP, Vol. 34, f. 31.

13. NP, Vol. 45, f. 129.

14. Katharine Gaskin, "Age at First Marriage in Europe Before 1850," Journal of Family History, Vol. 3 (1978), pp. 23-36.

15. Etienne Gautier and L. Henry, La population de Crulai Paroisse Normande (Paris, 1958), p. 84. E. A. Wrigley, "Family Limitation in Pre-Industrial England," Economic History Review, Vol. 29 (1966), p. 87.

16. Franklin F. Mendels, "Notes on the Age of Maternity, Population Growth and Family Structure in the Past," Journal of Family History, Vol. 3 (1978), pp. 236-250.

17. The marriage records of 1824 include a case of disguised paternity. Apparently an infant was born so soon after the parents' marriage that the husband doubted that he was the father. In the end husband and wife agreed to keep the dispute private and raised the child as legitimate. The true paternity was not made known until the son sought to marry the daughter of his biological father.

18. The estimate for Type C unions is slightly biased in specific instances although not as an average. It would now seem better to estimate the date of coupling by simply subtracting the average protogenesique interval of Type M unions from the date of the first prenuptially conceived birth, ignoring the marriage date altogether.

19. In the baptism book of 1825 the following signed statement appears: "I handed over this book and other things of this sort with the disorder in which I found them . . . ." The visit of the Archbishop in 1838 produced an immediate improvement in the celebration of sacraments and the administration of the parish books. Noting the last visitation had been in 1810, he ordered subsequent entries to be entered opportunely according to a model format under pain of severe penalty. Nevertheless, the marriage records were not organized carefully until 1854. From 1837 to 1847, there were 265 marriage acts lacking the corresponding nuptial testimonies and 84 testimonies with no record of a marriage. From 1854 to 1871 there were 5 and 23, respectively. From 1871 to 1896 there were only a few testimonies missing, all dated November 1890.

20. The downward bias in calculated age of marriage--inevitable for the first cohort of a reconstitution study where ages are derived from birth dates--is overcome here by not using linked birthdates unless the declared age at marriage is also known.

21. Estimates of Chilean population growth during the colonial era are not convincing. See McCaa "Chilean Social and," pp. 105-106. In an analysis of European growth rates in the eighteenth century, E. A. Wrigley (Population and History [New York, 1969], p. 152 and Table 5.1) reports only two regions with rates above 1 percent per year and one of these he characterizes as "suspiciously high."

22. MI, Vol. 317, f. 196.

23. GP, Vol. 1867, f. 52-53.

24. GP, Annual reports dated 1873, 1875, and 1879.

25. The differences could well lie within the range of error. The data are as follows:

TOTAL MARITAL FERTILITY RATES FOR PETORCA WOMEN BORN IN THE NINETEENTH CENTURY

	Female Birth Cohort				
	1800-19	1820-39	1840-59	1860-79	1880-94
Type M Unions					
Corrected rate	9.0	7.3	7.7	7.4	8.8
Estimated error (%)	35	18	7	3	0
N (at age 30-34)	73	94	76	61	26
Other Unions					
Corrected rate	9.4	8.3	9.2	8.8	8.6
Estimated error (%)	18	12	7	2	2
N (at age 30-34)	81	144	87	97	62

Dataset: Fertility.

NOTE: Fertility rates are for ages 20-44, women married at less than 30 years of age and excluding the age interval in which marriage occurred (to eliminate bias caused by prenuptial conceptions or births).

4
Fertility Change in Petorca

Where marriage and family constitute the social context of childbearing, age at marriage acts as an important cultural constraint on human reproduction. Nevertheless, historical demographers have discovered that cultural limits are broad and the range of fertility experiences great. The following material examines for the first time the natality history of a Chilean community.

The fertility of Petorca women has always been high, although on the whole never approaching an historical extreme. On the contrary, until recent decades Petorcans bore children at rates very similar to those of French and English village folk (Crulai and Colyton) prior to 1750. The greatest difference, higher fertility shortly after marriage, can be explained by the prevalence of prenuptial conceptions in Petorca and, beginning in 1930, the sharp rise in fecundability of teenage brides. Fertility differentials by age of marriage suggest a natural pattern of childbearing. Nevertheless, one subgroup shows strong parity-specific contraception practices also beginning in the 1930s. Fertility differentials, present in all cohorts from the 1840s, are small for conventional social variables (spouses' legitimacy, literacy, and occupation). Instead, prenuptial conception experience was the most important factor in differentiating marital fertility rates. Women with one or more prenuptial conceptions had significantly higher marital fertility than those without. Finally, refined examination of temporal variations reveals a temporary decline in fertility rates during the crisis decades 1860-1880.

The analysis of Chilean fertility suffers from three defects. First, fertility behavior prior to 1930 has been analyzed superficially with highly aggregated, general data. No recent scholar has attempted to go beyond crude rates or notoriously unreliable child-woman ratios. Second, fertility change since the 1930s has been the subject of more systematic analysis, but little work has been done toward describing or explaining regional or class differentials. Third, the failure to distinguish between marital and nonmarital fertility has been particularly unfortunate.[1] While the aggregate statistics certainly permit more extensive scrutiny than has been the case so far, the kind of data available, at least prior to 1930, is largely inadequate for studying Chilean fertility change in any detail. Age specific fertility data, one of the principal requisites for much natality analysis, was first published in 1911; tabulations of births by age and marital status were not prepared until 1930. Parity specific tables began only in 1952.[2]

FAMILY RECONSTITUTION AND THE SELECTION OF GENEALOGIES FOR THE STUDY OF FERTILITY

While Chile was a leader in Latin America in the publication of fertility data, nevertheless, because of the tardiness with which important series were begun, the historical evolution of Chilean fertility trends must be constructed through a reworking of the manuscript birth registers. The approach used here is that of family life histories, or family reconstitution. If the histories offer potentially rich analytical possibilities, they are not wholly satisfactory for two principal reasons. First, only a fraction of the family histories (28.2 percent in this instance) are analyzable because of technical requirements. Secondly, errors, biases, and mistakes inherent in the original data or introduced in the tedious compilation, linkage, and analytical stages create further difficulties.

A great number of family histories must be discarded as incomplete (Table 4.1). Since technical considerations limit the most sophisticated analysis to marital fertility, all histories lacking a marriage date, some 10,000, are thereby excluded. Moreover, marriages without an indication of the end of the marital union, that is the death date of the first spouse to die (or for families still intact in 1970, a probabilistic linkage with the 1970 census schedules), are also left aside. Slightly more than three-fifths of all marriages were rejected for this reason. A trivial number must be discarded for lack of the bride's date of birth (or age at some point). Furthermore, an examination of the resulting life histories by grooms' residence at marriage and birthplace indicated that even where all the customary inclusion criteria are fully satisfied, if the groom had a history of migration the fertility schedules all too frequently showed evidence of sporadic absences from the valley. Consequently, cases of this type--in which the groom was born outside of the valley or resided elsewhere at the time of the marriage--were excluded from the fertility dataset. The remaining histories, which correspond to family types M.I and M.II in the French system (except that here the geographically mobile are also excluded), include a greater proportion of the illiterate, the illegitimate, and those in farming occupations

TABLE 4.1
Selection of family histories for marital fertility analysis: Petorca, 1840-1969

Selection Criteria	N	Percent
Married, 1840-1969	5595	100.0
End of observation known	2211	39.5
Bride's age known	5273	94.2
Husband born in	3703	66.2
Husband resident in at marriage	5058	90.4
All criteria combined	1575	28.2

Comparison of Marriage and Fertility Datasets

Variable	Marriage Dataset (N)	Fertility Dataset (N)	Percent Included	Index
Total cases	5595	1575	28.2	100
Both spouses signed	1397	294	21.1	75
Both spouses legitimate	3194	719	22.5	80
Groom in farm occupation	2124	702	33.1	117
Bride's age--all	5273	1575	29.9	100
12-19	1122	324	28.9	97
20-24	1587	512	32.3	108
25-29	1344	420	31.2	104
30-34	568	168	29.6	99
35+	652	151	23.2	78

Datasets: Marriages and Fertility.

than for marriages as a whole. On the other hand, the exclusion criteria are more or less independent of the bride's age at marriage.

The structural similarities between the marriage and fertility datasets serve to highlight the particular character of the histories under study. While a very substantial portion of the population is not analyzable (the mobile, natural unions, and the like), given the almost total lack of historical information about Chilean fertility it is important to study the experience of any group possible. It should be emphasized that in the analysis of marital fertility even with respect to that of the valley itself there is a bias toward farmers, the more fertile women, the geographically stable, and the less educated.

NONMARITAL FERTILITY

Before analyzing the fertility experiences of the select population, illegitimate fertility should be examined briefly. Although nonmarital fertility and the life pattern of illegitimate natality is not reducible to demographic rates, nevertheless one can safely conclude that unmarried women in the Petorca Valley have always had lower fertility than married women. Most fertility histories of the single show comparatively few children. Only rarely did single women have more than five or six children and most had only one or two births. Single women married, migrated, or bore children only sporadically. The data on family formation patterns indicate that for most Petorca women, natural family life was simply a stage during which one or two children might be procreated, followed by married life or prolonged spinsterhood with sporadic and consequently largely sterile sexual encounters. The proportion of illegitimate children whose mothers are known to have married in the community at a later date sheds some light on this pattern (Table 4.2). From one-fourth to one-third of all illegitimate births occurred to women who later married in Petorca. Moreover, after 1925 when the Registration Bureau began to amend parents' marriage dates to birth inscriptions regardless of place or date of occurrence, an additional 7 percent of all illegitimate births occurred to women who subsequently married outside the study area. Consequently the proportion of legitimate births is probably much greater than the tediously reconstructed figures suggest. As many as 80 percent of all infants were legitimate during the earliest and latest periods, while less than 66 percent were during the first decades of the twentieth century. Most of that decrease is likely the result of couples' objections to civil marriage and registrars' refusals to inscribe offspring from religious unions as legitimate.

Some additional appreciation of nonmarital fertility can be obtained by analyzing illegitimacy in two ways: the

TABLE 4.2
Nonmarital fertility and later marriage

	Birth Periods			
	1840-1864	1865-1894	1895-1929	1930-1964
Total births	10,880	10,327	8,491	9,349
Percent mothers married	80.0	73.0	64.7	81.3
Illegitimate births	3,166	3,863	4,303	3,026
Percent of total	29.1	37.4	50.7	32.4
Mothers later married	985	1,071	1,211	1,071
Percent of illegitimate	31.1	27.7	28.1	35.4

Dataset: Births.

TABLE 4.3
Illegitimate births as a percent of all births by age of mother

	Birth Cohort				
Age of Mother	1885-1899	1900-1924	1925-1944	1945-1959	1960-1969
-19	28.6	34.4	22.5	23.9	31.8
20-24	20.5	31.9	17.4	15.8	17.4
25-29	13.2	22.6	13.4	13.8	14.8
30-34	9.7	17.8	9.9	12.2	11.9
35+	6.6	13.1	11.6	13.4	16.6
Known ages (%)	13.2	22.0	14.4	15.5	17.4
(N)	496	1003	567	618	448
All illegitimate (%)	28.1	35.2	22.3	16.9	18.4
(N)	1469	2074	1059	702	488

Dataset: Births.

percentage of illegitimate births for each mothers' age group (Table 4.3) and the distribution of bastards by single mothers' ages (Table 4.4). The almost total absence of age data for single mothers prior to 1885 necessarily restricts attention to the civil registration era. Both tables support the general conclusion that most illegitimate births were born by young women. In each Table, the highest proportion of illegitimate births is registered for women at the youngest ages. On the other hand it should be noted that for most periods at least 10 percent of all births (and sometimes considerably more) by women aged thirty and above are illegitimate. This indicates that at least some women who bore natural children married at relatively advanced ages, if at all. When the age distribution of single mothers is examined cross-sectionally almost one-third of the natural births belong to older women (aged thirty or more years) with only tiny variations from period to period.

Nevertheless, even this somewhat surprising percentage does not mean that illegitimate fertility rates were necessarily high, much less approaching that of legitimate unions. The two brief glimpses of total fertility for unmarried women derived from the census lists for 1865 and 1970 show that women who remained unmarried throughout the most fecund years, on the average fell very short of the levels attained by married women (Table 4.5). Both today and in the distant past, legal marriage greatly enhanced fertility. Furthermore, the differences would be even greater if single women without children were included in the figures. (The entries for married women include childless couples. In 1865 they accounted for some 10 percent of the total, but only 2 percent in 1970.) Both the census lists and the fertility histories suggest that while Petorca women began to bear children several years before reaching marriageable age, most of those who failed to marry at all typically entered a stage of markedly lower fertility as compared to the levels of married women. In the analysis which follows the fertility experience of women who never married in the study area is excluded from further scrutiny. On the other hand, for those who did marry in the valley, fertility histories both before and after marriage are analyzed.

FAULTY RECORDS

A second obstacle to ascertaining the fertility behavior of the valley's population is that of data quality. A more exhaustive treatment of this problem is presented in Appendix I; a summary of conclusions most pertinent for the analysis of marital fertility is presented here. In general Chilean vital statistics, particularly those on births, have been considered very unreliable, especially for earlier epochs. Nevertheless, analysis of births

TABLE 4.4
Illegitimate births by age of mother (in percentages)

			Birth Cohort		
Age of Mother	1885-1899	1900-1924	1925-1944	1945-1959	1960-1969
-19	16.1	11.9	19.8	24.8	23.4
20-24	29.2	29.8	27.5	23.1	23.2
25-29	25.6	25.5	23.5	18.9	20.3
30-34	16.1	18.1	12.9	14.9	13.6
35+	12.9	14.8	16.4	18.3	19.4
Total (%)	99.9	100.1	100.1	100.0	99.9
(N)	496	1003	567	618	448
Unknown (N)	973	1071	490	84	40
(%)	66.2	51.6	46.4	12.0	8.2

Dataset: Births.

TABLE 4.5
Fertility and marital status: Petorca, 1865, 1970

	1865 CENSUS MANUSCRIPTS			
	35-44		45-54	
	Married	Single Mothers	Married	Single Mothers
Mean children listed	4.12	2.00	4.00	1.73
No. of women	77	16	44	11
	1970 CENSUS LISTS			
	35-44		45+	
	Married	Single Mothers	Married	Single Mothers
Mean children ever born	6.90	4.50	7.10	5.22
No. of women	122	12	148	9

Sources: Censo de Petorca de 1865. 1970 lists provided by the National Statistical Institute.

NOTE: For method of elaboration see Appendix II.

TABLE 4.6
Rate of birth omissions: Petorca 1840-1969

	SELECT FERTILITY HISTORIES			
	Parent's Marriage Period			
Birth Events	1840-1862	1863-1894	1895-1929	1930-1969
Omissions	66	60	19	5
Death inscriptions	419	565	455	105
Percent omitted	15.8	10.6	4.2	4.8
Born after parent's marriage				
Omissions (N)	52	51	8	3
Omissions (%)	13.4	9.9	2.2	3.5
	REJECTED FERTILITY HISTORIES			
Omissions	64	96	33	18
Death inscriptions	246	696	303	158
Percent omitted	26.0	13.8	9.8	11.4

Dataset: Marriages.

NOTE: "Omissions" indicate the number of individuals who died at age one or older and for whom no birth registration was located. "Death inscriptions" make up the total child and adult deaths (i.e. excluding deaths to infants aged less than one year) for offspring of the specified family type. Fleury and Henry (1958, pp. 48-52) estimate omissions from offspring who later married (yielded an error rate of 2-4 percent for Crulai parish, 1674-1742). Deaths are used here to avoid the problem caused by abrupt termination of the study (few people born after 1950 married before 1970) and by the confusion resulting from the change to civil marriage at the end of the last century. The two indicators produce nearly identical results except for the recent period (as they do for Crulai also).

registered in the Petorca Valley shows that the coverage was surprisingly complete in the nineteenth century (if very poor in comparison to the completeness of certain European registers), and for legitimate children reached respectable levels by the beginning of this century. In fact, birth registration is best for families precisely selected for intensive study (Table 4.6).

Apparently, an identifiable subset of families has been integrated into the national registration system, whether ecclesiastical or civil, for over a century and it is precisely this group whose marital fertility histories are analyzable according to the rules of family

TABLE 4.7
Known birth registration omissions by type of error: Petorca, 1840-1969

	Marriage Periods (of parents)			
Source of Omission	1840-1862	1863-1894	1895-1929	1930-1969
Temporary absence (%)	2.8	3.7	1.1	0
Failure to register (%)	10.6	6.2	1.1	3.5
Total omissions (N)	52	51	8	3
Total omissions (%)	13.4	9.9	2.2	3.5

Dataset: Fertility.

NOTE: For explanations of estimating procedures see Table 4.6. Percentages refer to births occurring after marriage for select families.

reconstitution. The rate of omissions for rejected families is usually 50 percent greater than that of prime families. Nevertheless, when compared with coverage in some eighteenth-century French parishes omissions are two, three, and even four times higher in the Petorca Valley.[3]

The quality of birth registration coverage for family reconstitution purposes is determined by two factors: the failure to inscribe a birth, and temporary absences from the registration area when a birth occurs, which consequently is registered elsewhere. Because of the consistent recording of birthplace information in the Petorca registers, it is possible to clearly differentiate between the two sources of error with some confidence. In contrast to French parish studies, where temporary absences are presumed to account for most of the birth omissions, in the Petorca Valley the failure to register births has been and continues to be the principal source of omissions (Table 4.7). Perhaps the most surprising trend is the apparent deterioration in registration efficiency for recent decades. Although the estimate for the latest period is derived from only three omissions, it is possible that the trend is a real one. The delay in registering legitimate births has increased substantially since 1940. More detailed data on registration errors by marriage cohorts and wives' birth cohorts show a steady improvement from the very high levels of the mid-nineteenth century through 1930 (Figure 4.1).

Fertility measures presented below are adjusted for estimated rates of birth omissions specific for the respective cohort. Where special subsets are analyzed, adjustments for the time period and appropriate category

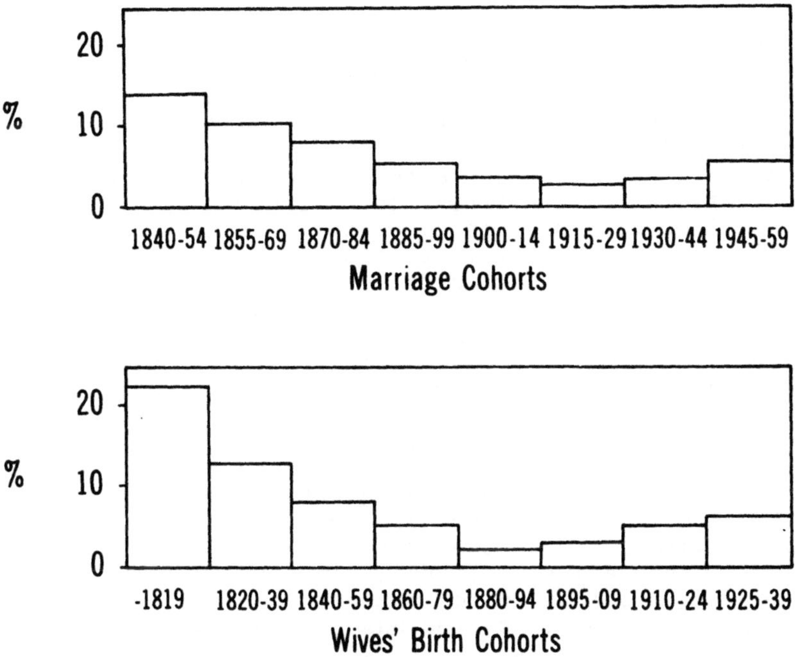

Dataset: Fertility

Figure 4.1 Birth omissions by marriage cohorts and wives' birth cohorts: select families, Petorca Valley

(occupation, literacy, etc.) are also reported. Nevertheless, with few exceptions, period effects overshadow social and demographic effects (Table 4.8). Successively disaggregated adjustments (period, age at marriage, age at risk, and some social variable) cannot be made because the absolute number of omissions is too few to permit minutely detailed corrections.

As a further cautionary note, it should be apparent that the level of confidence in the figures reported here is related to the level of aggregation. The disturbing effects of random variation and small numbers increase with each level of refinement; therefore, only very great differences in adjusted fertility rates between periods or social groups suffice to arouse much conviction that perceived differences are true ones. Moreover the effects of the most important sources of error (temporary absences and failure to register) is to underestimate actual fertility levels. In other words, observed fertility estimates must be considered absolute minima. The corrected figures are probably nearer the real fertility levels than raw, unadjusted ones. However, once corrections are made it is possible that the adjusted figures are either too high or still too low. The relative magnitude of the correction factors might be considered a reliable indicator of the degree of confidence with which specific estimates may be analyzed. As a concrete quantitative guideline, one might guess that the actual levels are likely to lie somewhere within a band the width of the error rate and centered on the adjusted figure. In summary, what follows must be understood as approximations, derived through a systematic chain of reasoning based on presuppositions which, if all the facts were known, would not always be correct.

MARITAL AND NATURAL FERTILITY, 1840-1969

The fertility levels of the Petorca Valley show a remarkable stability over the past one hundred thirty years (Figure 4.2). If the pace of childbearing has nudged downward at one generation or increased modestly for another, in the aggregate, neither the level nor the pattern of fertility has changed much. The outstanding characteristics of natality in the Petorca Valley are the high level and the convex shape of the fertility curve. Clearly this is a natural fertility regime, as opposed to a population practicing birth control (Figure 4.3). The Petorcan pattern for women marrying 1895-1929 is almost identical to that of two widely cited European natural fertility populations: sixteenth-century Colyton (England) and eighteenth-century Crulai (France). It is not surprising that Petorca women were less prolific than French Canadian women in the eighteenth century, since the latter are regarded as approaching the biological maximum for human

TABLE 4.8
Birth registration omissions by marriage periods and social groups: Petorca, 1840-1969 (percent)

Variable (relates to spouses)	Marriage Period 1840-1862	1863-1894	1895-1929	1930-1969
Total omissions	13.4	7.6	2.2	3.5
Legitimate				
Both	13.8	8.4	3.5	2.5
Other	12.7	5.9	1.0	4.4
Literate				
Both	0	9.4	4.5	2.6
Other	13.8	7.4	1.7	4.3
Occupation				
Farmer	16.8	7.5	2.4	4.2
Other	11.9	7.6	1.5	0
Women's age at risk of childbearing*				
15-19	20.8	15.4	0	0
20-24	13.3	12.0	4.4	7.7
25-29	9.4	5.8	3.9	5.5
30-34	13.0	8.2	2.1	0
Women's age at marriage*				
15-19	12.6	9.9	2.1	5.9
20-24	12.9	7.0	1.8	3.3
25-29	9.5	9.6	2.9	5.6
30-39	13.0	13.3	2.7	0
Years elapsed since marriage (wife's marriage age less than 30 years)				
Before marriage	41.5	25.7	13.4	18.2
0-4 years	17.6	5.5	2.4	5.0
5-9	10.6	9.2	1.4	0
10-14	13.1	9.7	0	0
15-19	21.1	3.9	0	0
Family beginnings*				
Marriage	10.1	6.4	0	0
Premarital conception	13.1	14.1	3.0	4.4

Dataset: Fertility.

NOTE: All percentages refer to known omissions after spouse's marriage except for the single "before marriage" estimate. Groups marked with an asterisk refer only to women marrying before age 40 and at risk through age 44. Other groups refer to births of all women in Fertility Dataset.

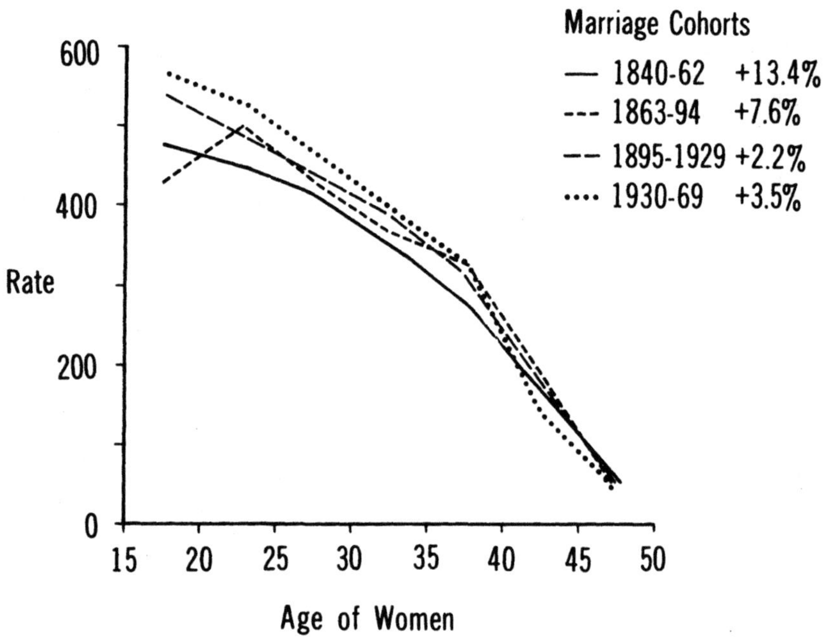

Dataset: Fertility

Figure 4.2 Age-specific marital fertility: Petorca Valley, 1840-1969

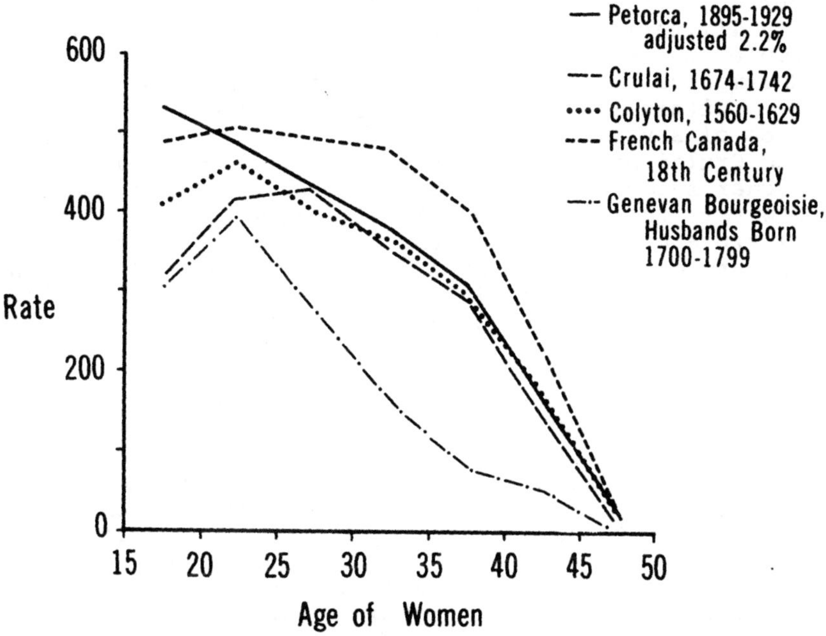

Sources: Fertility Dataset; Gautier and Henry (1958), p. 101; Wrigley (1967), p. 89; Henripin (1954), p. 60; Henry (1956), p. 76.

Figure 4.3 Natural and controlled fertility: examples from five historical populations

populations.

The shape of all natural fertility curves are remarkably similar: a convex, bulging outward pattern typical of couples who do not consciously restrict childbearing to an individually desired or collectively prescribed number of offspring. In contrast the Genevan Bourgeoisie fertility curve is concave, reflecting the effects of conscious family limitation notable from age thirty onward. This example is one of the earliest cases of fertility control documented by family reconstitution analysis.

Within the natural fertility group, the sole difference of any significance between Petorca on the one hand and Crulai and Colyton on the other is the relatively higher rates at younger ages in the Chilean community. However, this exceptionally high fertility is almost wholly explained by the greater incidence of pregnant brides. The proportion has always been very great, fluctuating in a narrow range from 24 to 31 percent (see Table 3.11) versus less than 3 and 22 percent for Crulai and Colyton respectively.[4]

NATALITY RATES OF YOUNG BRIDES

The exclusion of pregnant brides from the Petorca rates leaves little doubt about the main reason for fertility variations at young ages from one cohort to another (Figure 4.4). The fertility rate for brides aged 20-24 who were not pregnant at marriage not only remains constant for three of the four broad marriage cohorts, but is also surprisingly close to the corresponding figure for Crulai. The figures for this age group suggest that biological fecundability in the Petorca Valley has varied little over the past hundred years. An increase possibly occurred around the middle of the nineteenth century, although estimates for the early cohorts are too insecure to place much confidence in the observed difference.

On the other hand, the fertility rate for pregnant brides aged 20-24 is not only greater for each cohort but is much more variable as well. Their fertility rates are especially sensitive to changing social customs with respect to pregnancy as a stimulus to marry. During some periods pregnant brides were more apt to give birth soon after the wedding day, while at other times marriage was more likely to occur very soon after the pregnancy was discovered. The fertility rate immediately after marriage is consequently artificially inflated or dampened according to the severity of the change. Overall fertility variations for this age group is explained primarily by fluctuations in the relative frequency of brides with prenuptial conceptions and the interim between marriage and the birth of a prenuptially conceived infant.

Teen brides on the other hand show important biological changes in fecundability. In recent decades teen

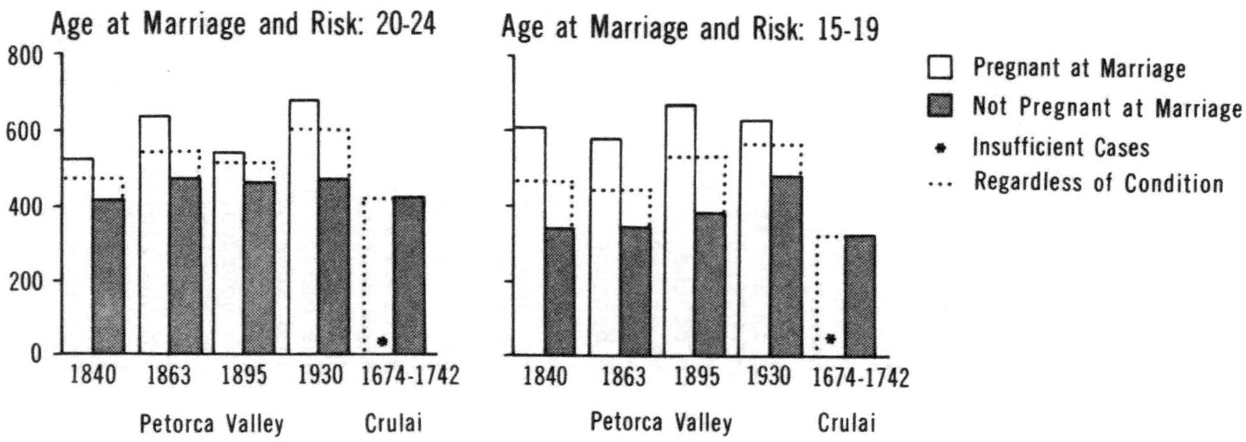

Sources: Fertility Dataset; Gautier and Henry, p. 101.

Note: Error rates as reported in Table 4.8.

Figure 4.4 Fertility by pregnancy condition of brides: Petorca Valley, 1840-1969

brides not pregnant at marriage bore considerably more children during their first years of marriage than earlier generations (Figure 4.5). In fact, teenage subfecundity, normally found in reconstitution studies, disappears almost completely in Petorca after 1930. Now the fertility rates for young brides not pregnant at marriage are the same, whether they marry in their teens or twenties. The age of menarche very likely declined to such an extent that adolescent sterility is confined to the very early ages (less than fifteen years) and does not extend into the late teens to the degree that it did for earlier generations. A century ago the fertility rate for this group was barely greater than that for Crulai. Toward the end of the last century, the rate rose rather abruptly and continued to slowly increase for about fifty years; however, until 1910 much of the change is explained by the increasing proportion of older teen brides rather than rising fecundability. For the last three cohorts the surge in fertility are real and even more impressive than depicted in the chart because the average age of teen brides simultaneously declined by a full year. For recent cohorts the rate is over 40 percent greater than a century and a half ago. The decline in age at marriage and the biological increase in fecundability for teenagers have substantial implications for both the size of individual families and the growth rate of the valley. On the average the completed family size of teen brides, if there were no adjustments in fecundity at later ages, would have increased by about one child because of the youthfulness of brides and their earlier age at marriage.

The fertility rates of pregnant teen brides show comparatively little change over time. The rates for this group have always been extremely high. They can hardly be compared with those of other ages because the denominator of the rate (women years in observation) is severely underestimated through the elimination of time actually at risk prior to marriage. For brides aged 15-19 much of the time actually pregnant preceded marriage and a greater proportion of the period of post-partum amenorrhea overlapped into the succeeding age group (20-24).

In summary, at the younger ages of motherhood, variation over time in marital fertility rates in the Petorca Valley derives mainly from two sources, one social and the other biological. The largest absolute change is social, but to some extent this is an artifact reflecting changing predispositions with regard to the timing of pregnancy and marriage. If the biologically induced variations are confined principally to the modern era and a single age group, they are nevertheless very important, particularly for understanding the course of fertility during the dynamic stages of the demographic transition.

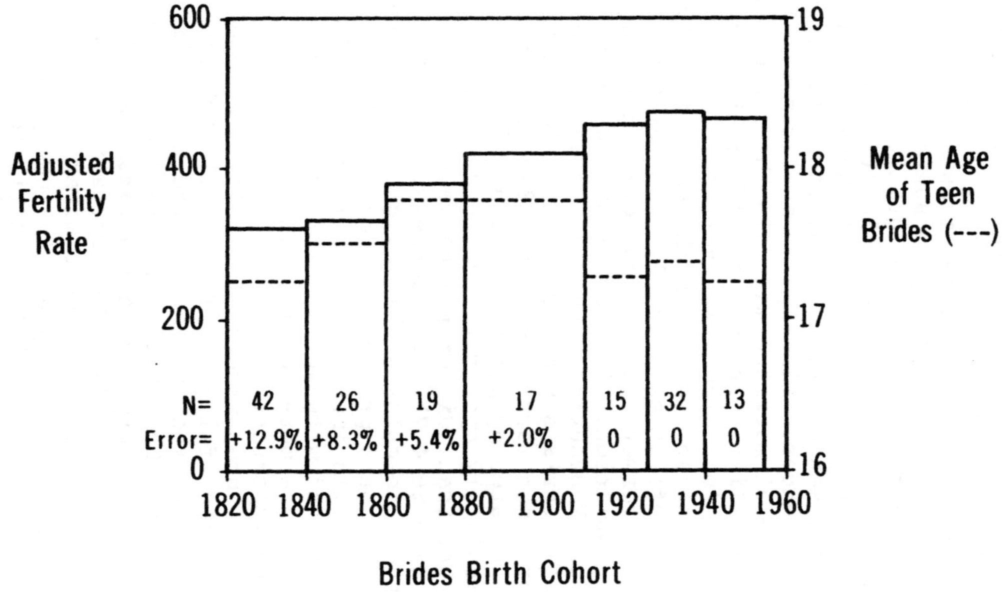

Dataset: Fertility

Figure 4.5 Fertility of not pregnant teen brides at age 15-19: Petorca Valley

FERTILITY PATTERNS BY AGE AT MARRIAGE

Fertility rates by age at marriage for the population as a whole also indicate a natural fertility regime for all periods studied (Figure 4.6). In general the differences in fertility rates from age thirty and above are minor. It has long been argued that the lack of fertility differentials by age at marriage is an indication of natural fertility.[5] While the relevant curves for the Petorca Valley are not exactly identical, the variations do not indicate birth control for at least three reasons. In the first place, most of the deviations beyond age twenty-nine are absolutely small. Secondly, the poor quality of the data suggests caution. One might expect slightly lower fertility rates for women marrying early if there were a direct relationship between duration of marriage and likelihood of temporary absences. Finally, in most cases, all the curves for each age at marriage maintain the convexity typical of natural fertility populations. After 1862 the slope of the legitimate fertility curve for women marrying in their teens shows a steep decline in the early twenties, followed by a leveling off at ages 30-39. The relatively dampened rates for the former group is not characteristic of a contracepting population. A study of an eighteenth-century French parish, Tourouvre au Perche, reveals duration of marriage differentials similar to those for Petorca, particularly for women married between 1840-1862 and 1895-1969.[6] Rates inflated by prenuptial conceptions for the age at risk immediately upon marriage in Petorca constitute the only significant difference between the two fertility patterns (Figure 4.7). Charbonneau, the author of the Tourouvre study, speculates that slight age at marriage differentials may be a product of a gradual increase in temporary sterility with increasing family size.[7] Temporary absences associated with age at marriage (women marrying at young ages are more apt to move about after marriage) may also be important.

The temporal charts presented so far suffer to some extent from an aggregation fallacy. The social structure of the valley has been undergoing change since the earliest days of its founding. Education has spread widely to all classes during this century. Bastardy rates have waxed and waned over long periods. The occupational structure of the valley has slowly become more diversified since the middle of the past century and the occupational elite increased in relative size at least until the beginning of this century. Finally, and most important, social pressure to legitimize family unions (and thereby qualify for analysis here) has varied considerably from one epoch to another. Aggregated fertility rates indicate the sum experience of a particular generation, but as the structural composition of the whole shifts, fertility rates must be disaggregated to determine differences produced by changing social structure and by varying fertility

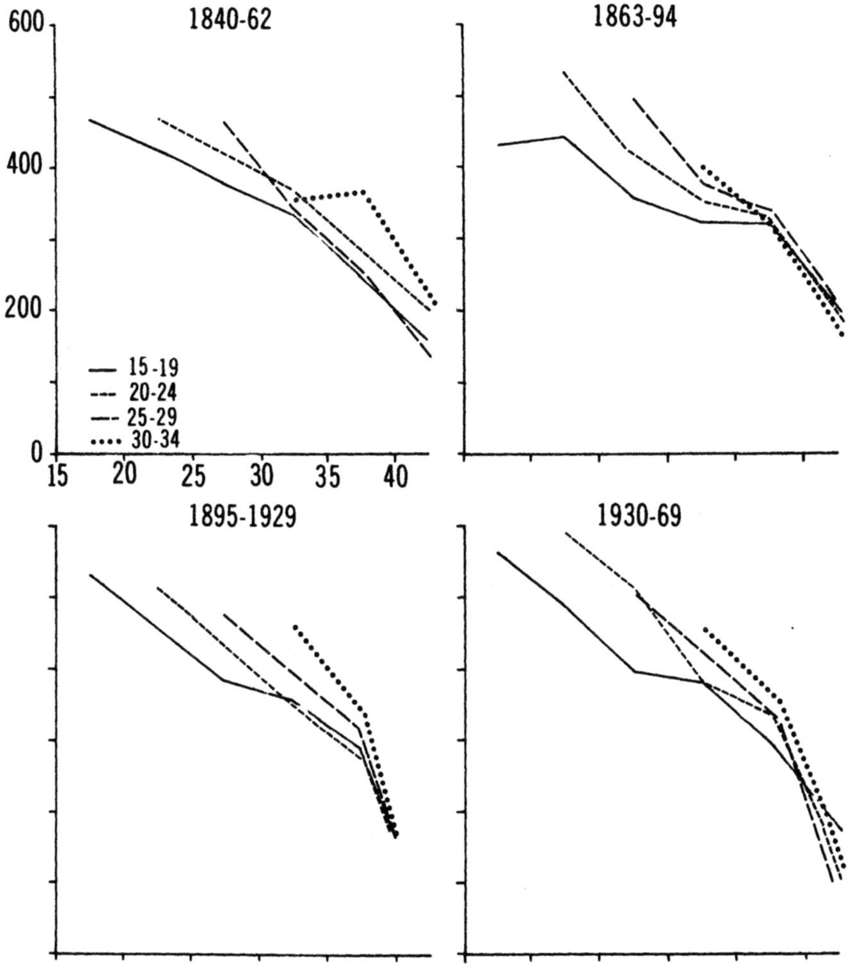

Dataset: Fertility

Note: Correction factors as reported in Table 4.8.

Figure 4.6 Legitimate fertility by age at marriage for marriage cohorts: Petorca, 1840-1969

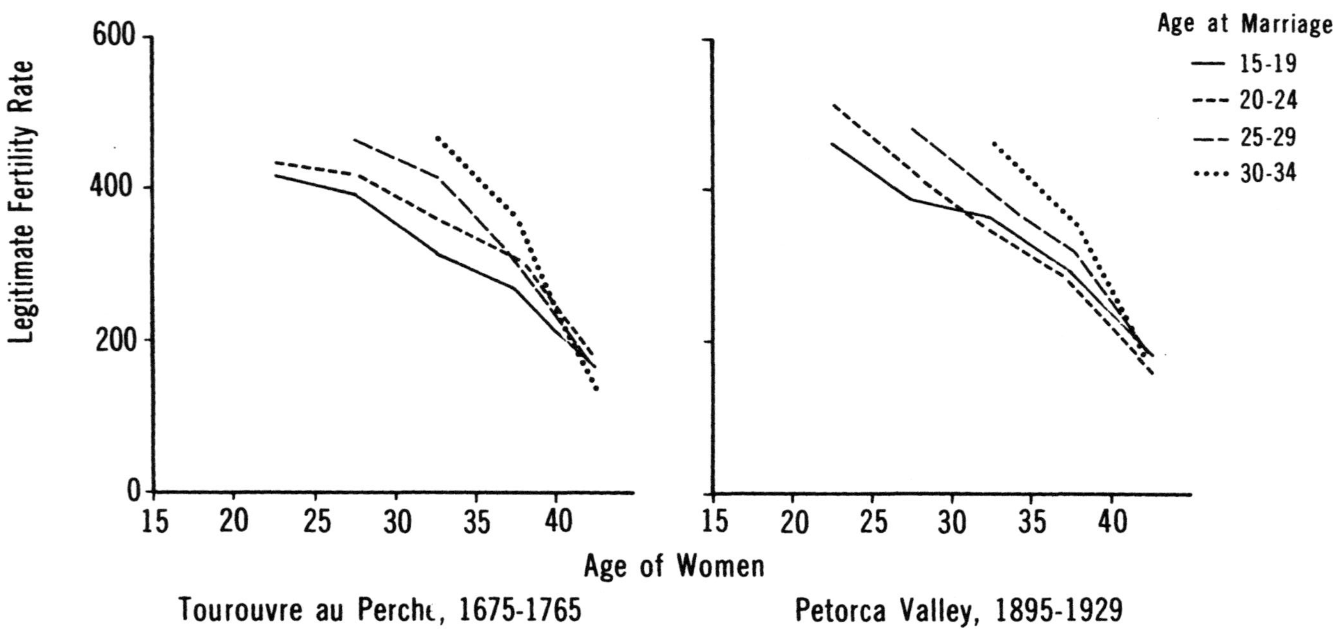

Sources: Fertility Dataset; Charbonneau, p. 100.

Figure 4.7 Age at marriage fertility differentials from two family reconstitution studies

behavior.

Two elements of natality change are important here: fertility levels and the shape of the fertility curve. Four social variables, introduced earlier in the discussion of marriage patterns, are useful for controlling the effects of structural variations from period to period: (1) manner of initiating the family union (some premarital conceptions or none); (2) husband's occupation (farming or nonfarming); (3) ability of spouses to sign the marriage register (both signed or other); and (4) legitimacy of spouses as indicated in the marriage act (both legitimate or other).

ASSOCIATION BETWEEN PRENUPTIAL CONCEPTIONS AND MARITAL FERTILITY

Prenuptial conception experience is the single most important social determinant of fertility in each period in terms of both the absolute magnitude of differentials and maximum statistical heterogeneity (Table 4.9). The largest fertility differences are found when the dataset is divided according to family initiation type, and the cases are thereby bifurcated into more or less equal groups. Fertility rates at all ages for women with some prenuptial conceptions are always 10 to 20 percent higher than those for women with no premarital conceptions. Moreover there is never less than 40 nor more than 60 percent of the cases in either of the groups. If occupational differentials are of the same magnitude, the division of the fertility histories by occupation produces two groups of very unequal size. When occupational designations are systematic (after 1895), over 80 percent of the histories are for farmers and only 20 percent for nonfarmers. Literacy also seems to account for much variation at least during two periods, but the dataset is highly homogeneous (most women in one group) with respect to educational experience. When fertility differences are great, the split is lopsided; and, when the histories divide into relatively equal groups of signing and not-signing, the fertility differences are trivial. Finally, the legitimacy variable consistently maximizes heterogeneity of cases but only tiny fertility differences result.

As an analytical variable, prenuptial conception experience has several attractive features which are lacking with the other social variables. Premarital sexual relations are systematically related with occupation, literacy, and legitimacy. A higher proportion of literate spouses began family life with marriage. Likewise, brides from petite bourgeois families overwhelmingly married first and then began bearing children. But for most years both of these groups made up only a tiny sliver of the entire social structure. On the other hand, in each period a significant portion of couples began their families first and

TABLE 4.9
Fertility differentials and distribution of cases: Petorca, 1840-1969

Variable	Percentage Difference in Total Fertility Rate Ages 20-44				Percentage of Women in Category at Ages 30-34				
	1840	1863	1895	1930	Category	1840	1863	1895	1930
Prenuptial conceptions	14	20	13	20	Some	53.9	41.9	58.7	52.7
Husband's occupation	7	23	19	14	Farming	31.6	47.4	80.4	78.6
Spouses' signature	-18	0	-12	-3	Both signed	4.7	9.7	27.7	55.5
Spouses' legitimacy	-6	2	-9	-2	Both legitimate	57.2	68.9	50.2	56.2
Total fertility rate (ages 20-44)	8.12	9.18	8.98	9.31	Total cases	297	289	271	281

Dataset: Fertility.

NOTE: The percentage difference in total fertility rate indicates how much the two categories of each variable differ from one another. For example, in 1840 marriages in which both spouses signed produced a total fertility rate eighteen percent lower than marriages in which at least one spouse did not sign. Rates for prenuptial conception history do not include data for the age group in which the marriage occurred. Distribution of families by occupation prior to 1895 is misleading because of the relatively large number for which no occupation was specified.

then married. Simply the chronological order of these two events determined subsequent marital fertility better than any other variable. Biological fecundability, attitudes about sexuality and intercourse, social nuances more subtle than occupation, literacy, or legitimacy, and at some date family size preferences--all are interwoven in this variable.

Differentials in fertility levels by prenuptial conception experience are striking for each period (Figure 4.8). The fertility differences at all ages usually amount to at least 10 percent and are often 20 percent or more. The experiential differences are even greater than reported here because fertility immediately after marriage is excluded in order to reduce aberrations caused by prenuptial conceptions. While the curves are obviously systematically related, nevertheless, women without premarital conceptions always had lower fertility than those with. Moreover the relative differences are almost always greater at ages thirty and above. Does this suggest that a sizeable group of Petorcans were consciously limiting their fertility in the nineteenth century? The numerical argument is based on a few cases and the literary evidence nil; however, it should be remembered that marriages after 1863 show demographic evidence of a malthusian preventive response to population pressure (delayed marriage and greater proportions never marrying; see Chapter 3). It is also likely that single women who became pregnant were less apt to legally marry than in any other period. This fact may help explain the very great differences in fertility levels for the two groups in this period. The mating and marriage process operated to concentrate the more fecund in one group and the less fecund in the other. Consequently, the evidence for conscious fertility limitation within marriage is weak. The only ages at which the curve bears any semblance to a malthusian one are twenty-five to twenty-nine, and that dip could be erased by minor corrections. Probably more important is that there is no relationship between age at marriage and fertility at thirty years and beyond (Table 4.10). Differences are small; the required inverse correlation is weak and inconsistent. Finally, cumulative fertility from age thirty is actually higher for this group than at other periods.

EFFECTS OF SOCIAL STATUS

Occupation is the second most important variable in terms of the magnitude of fertility differences between groups and the proportion of cases in each category (Figure 4.9). Farming families at every age and period almost invariably had higher fertility than nonfarmers. By 1863 the differences are both well established and large (about 20 percent). Notably, farmers clearly had very high fertility at all dates. Nevertheless, the differences between

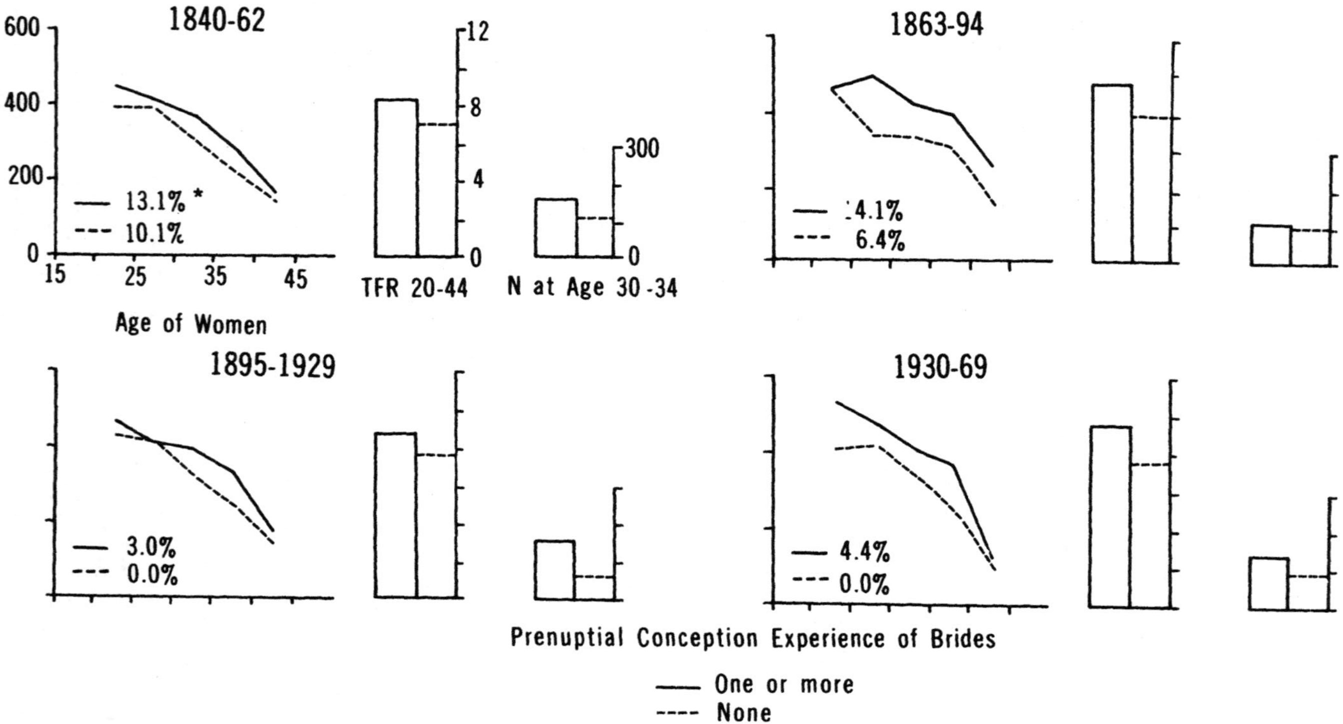

*correction for omissions

Dataset: Fertility

Figure 4.8 Fertility differentials by bride's premarital conception history

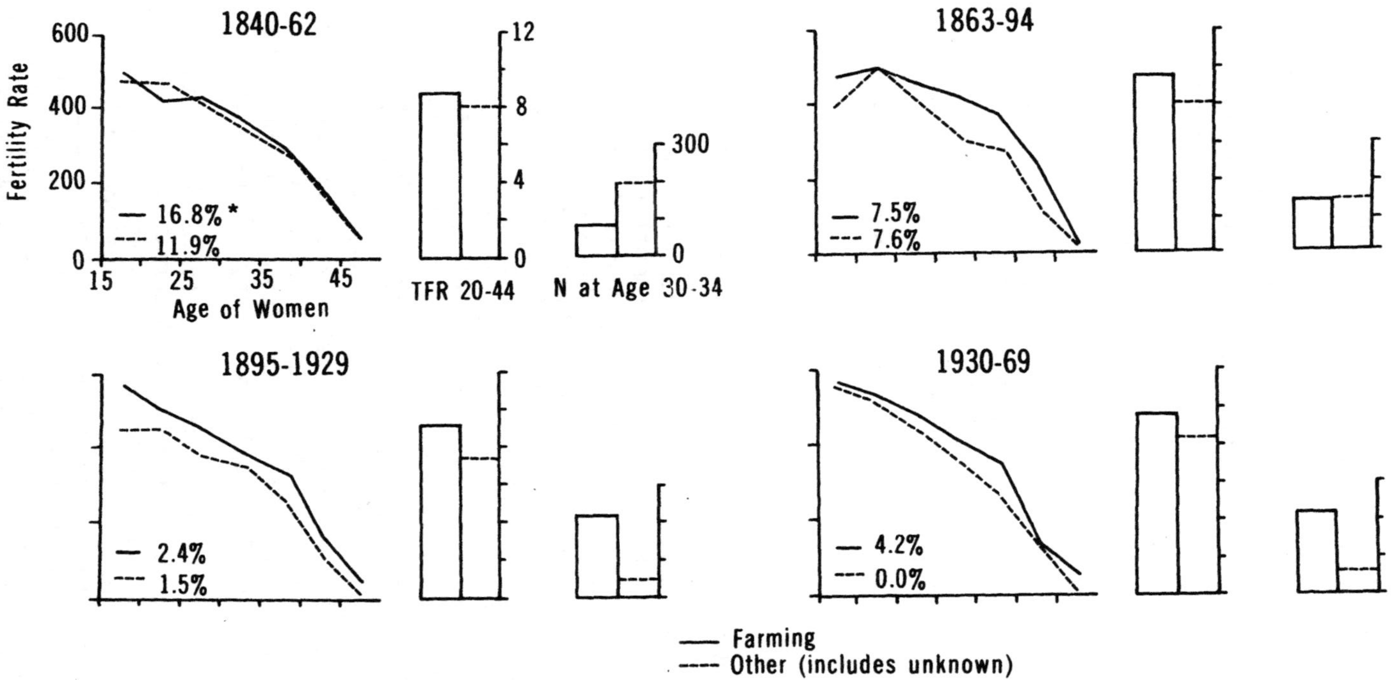

*correction for omissions

Dataset: Fertility

Figure 4.9 Fertility differentials according to occupation of husband

TABLE 4.10
Cumulative fertility rates for ages 30-44 by age at marriage and prenuptial conception experience, 1840-1969

	Marriage Period			
Age at Marriage	1840-1862	1863-1894	1895-1929	1930-1969
No premarital conceptions				
15-19	3.42	3.86	3.80	3.28
20-24	3.88	3.71	3.84	3.53
25-29	2.74	4.07	3.13	3.88
Some premarital conceptions				
15-19	3.73	4.84	4.41	4.81
20-24	4.43	5.24	3.93	4.71
25-29	4.14	5.14	4.92	4.42

Dataset: Fertility.

NOTE: Figures indicate average children born according to marital fertility rates from ages 30 through 44.

farmers and nonfarmers are smaller than those by prenuptial pregnancy experience.

Fertility differentials according to the education of spouses are even smaller and less important (Figure 4.10). While the customary inverse relationship between education and fertility is present in the Petorca data, the extreme homogeneity of the married population means that the overall fertility levels are hardly affected by this variable. Moreover, prior to 1895, the number of educated couples was so small that little confidence can be placed in the estimates for this group. After 1895, the differential is systematic, but still small. Moreover, it is apparent that the major difference associated with prenuptial experiences is explained hardly at all by education.

The final set of rates, for spouses according to their legitimacy status at marriage, show trivial differences indeed (Figure 4.11). While the legitimate group usually had lower fertility than couples from illegitimate backgrounds, error could easily swamp any of these relationships.

The overall pattern of fertility differentials demonstrates that the most important determinant of marital fertility levels is prenuptial pregnancy history. Women who became pregnant before marrying systematically had higher marital fertility rates than those who did not. Both social and biological forces must have operated to produce these patterns. Prenuptial pregnancy perhaps stands as an indicator of sexual compatability, frequency

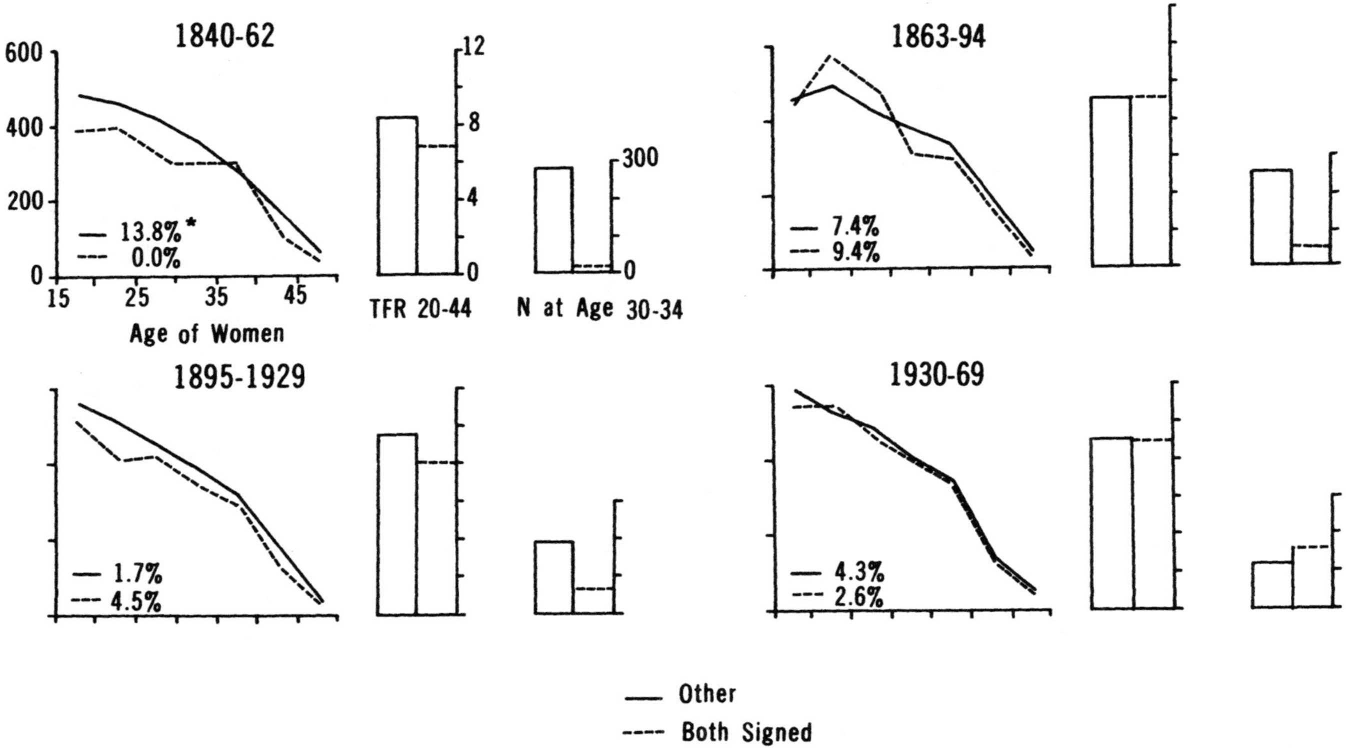

*correction for omissions

Dataset: Fertility

Figure 4.10 Fertility differentials by spouses' ability to sign name

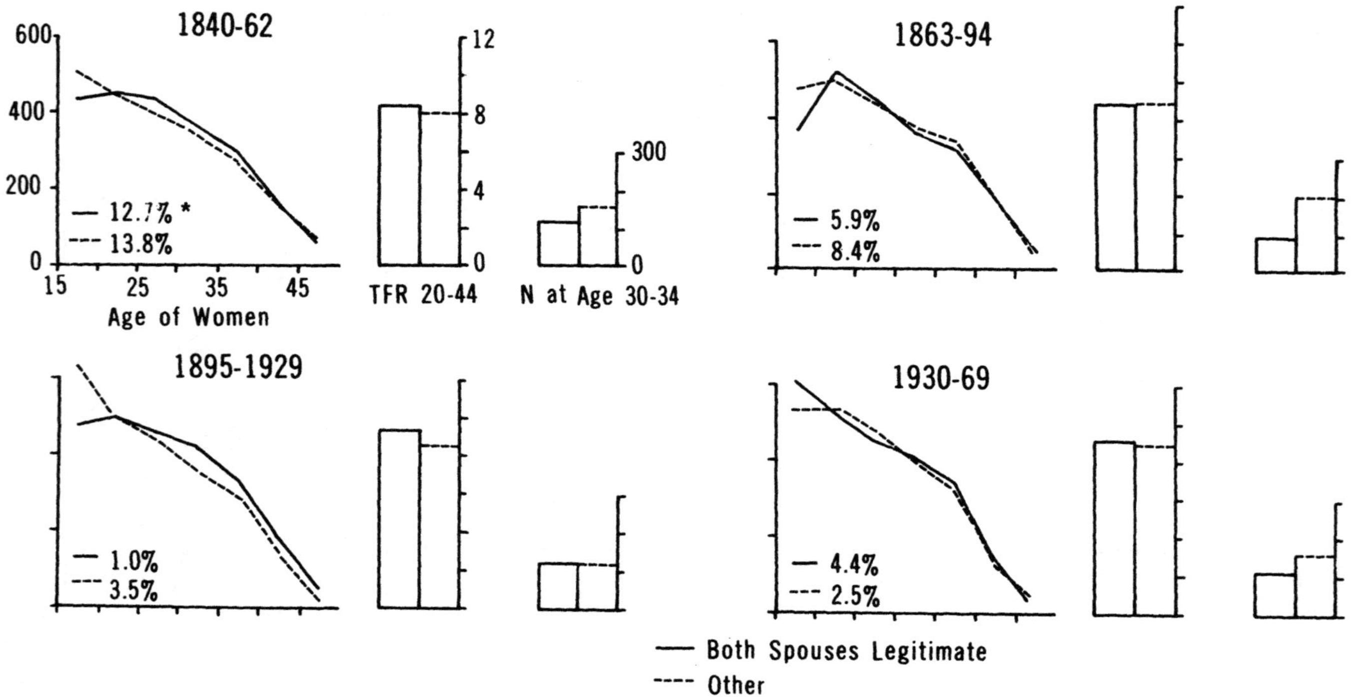

*corrections for omissions

Dataset: Fertility

Figure 4.11 Fertility differentials according to legitimacy of spouses

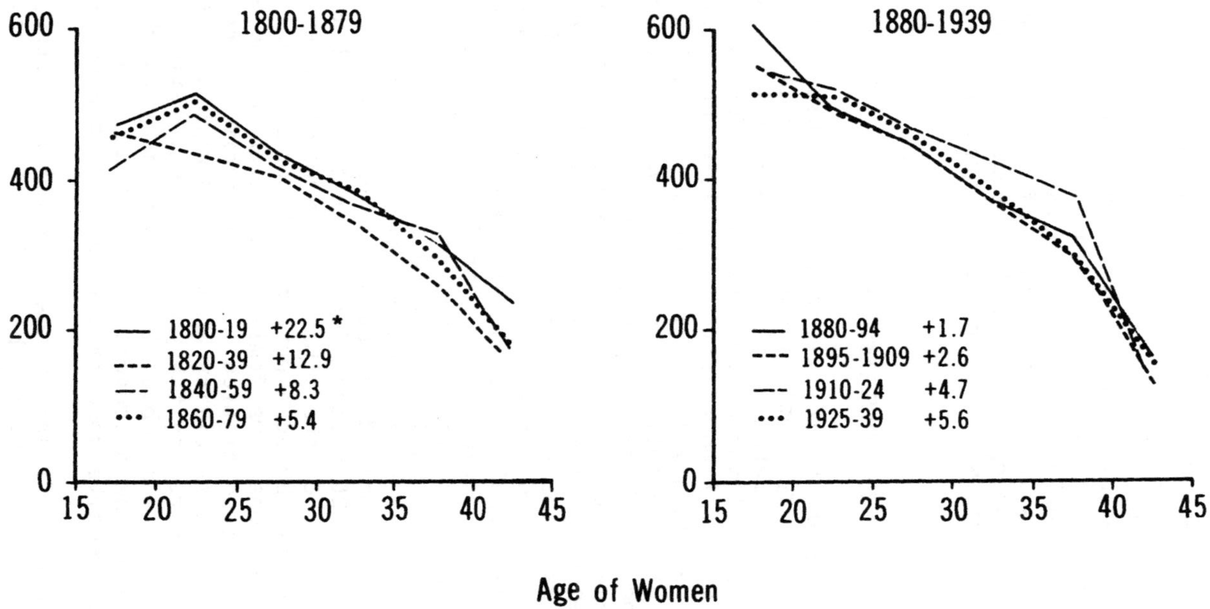

*correction for omissions

Dataset: Fertility

Figure 4.12 Marital fertility rates by women's birth cohort

of intercourse, preference for children, and strictly biological fecundability as well as class and culture. It is impossible to disentangle the various factors to weigh the importance of one relative to another. What is important is that the achievement of fertile sexual activity before marriage or vice-versa was strongly associated with subsequent natality rates.

To sum up, the level and shape of the aggregated fertility curves show only minor differences from one period to another. Measurable variations are generally associated with fluctuations in the proportion of brides experiencing prenuptial conceptions and their subsequent fertility. Rates for women who had prenuptial pregnancies show tiny variations.

DEMOGRAPHIC CRISIS AND FERTILITY DECLINE

The grouping of the fertility data into broad periods obscures two temporary fluctuations: one short-lived and episodic; the other transitional and secular (Figure 4.12). The first substantial variation over time in fertility levels is observed for women born 1820-1839; the second occurred about a century later, for women born 1910-1924. The fertility decline noted for the first birth cohort is too great to be attributed to problems of measurement. This is the same group of women who delayed marriage in the face of demographic crisis beginning in 1863. The total fertility rate for this cohort drops to 8.0, while all other cohorts are very close to or above 9.0. The decline occurred for all social groups and for each age at marriage; however, the decrease for poor families (i.e. uneducated farmers of illegitimate backgrounds) is twice that of other groups (Table 4.11). The fertility of poor women, which for other cohorts was always considerably above average, just barely surpassed the mean for this cohort. Poor women experienced a 20 percent decline in the total marital fertility rate. On the other hand, women with no premarital conceptions showed a more modest contraction. Once again, no hint of conscious family limitation can be elicited from any of these figures. Instead there occurred a general dampening of fertility at all ages with the largest declines registered by the poorest women. Given the type of information available, the mechanism by which this was achieved cannot be discovered. Nor is it apparent why fertility of successive cohorts returned to more normal levels.

The second significant change in fertility rates, a two-phased process marking the beginning of the transition to a modern fertility regime in the Petorca Valley, is discussed in the following chapter.

TABLE 4.11
Fertility decline in the nineteenth century: Petorca women born 1800-1859

	Women's Birth Cohort		
Total Fertility Rate	1800-1819	1820-1839	1840-1859
Ages 20-44	9.35	8.00	8.94
Percentage difference in TFR			
Ages 20-44	+17	8.00	+12
Poor	+17	8.29	+23
Women with prenuptial conceptions	+18	8.72	+16
Women without prenuptial conceptions	+21	6.88	+12

Dataset: Fertility.

NOTES

1. Sadie, "Población y mano," pp. 17-20. See also the study by Jorge Vidal, "Encuesta demográfica de Cauquenes: Estudio de la fecundidad," in Chile (Santiago, 1969), pp. 225-253; based on a survey in 1965 the author examines rural-urban and class differentials with no controls for marital status. Odette Tacla Chamy (Panorama Demográfico de Chile y su evolución en el presente siglo [Santiago, 1975], pp. 14-17) presents basic data for recent years.

2. See the respective Statistical Annuals.

3. Etienne Gautier and Louis Henry, La Population de Crulai Paroisse Normande (Paris, 1958), pp. 48-51; Charbonneau, Tourouvre-au-Perche, pp. 27-29.

4. Gautier and Henry, La population de, p. 135. E. A. Wrigley, "Family Limitation in Pre-Industrial England," Economic History Review, Vol. 29 (1966), pp. 88, note 2.

5. Louis Henry, "Some Data on Natural Fertility," Eugenics Quarterly, Vol. 8 (1961), pp. 81-91. The method recently developed by J. Dupaquier and M. Lachiver, in "Sur les debuts de la contraception en France ou les deux malthusianismes," Annales, E. S. C., Vol. 24 (1969), pp. 1391-1406, cannot be applied here because of the problem of birth underregistration.

6. Charbonneau, Tourouvre-au-Perche, pp. 101-102.

7. Ibid.

5
The Demographic Transition in the Petorca Valley

In its classic formulation, the demographic transition is schematized as a four-stage process (Figure 5.1).[1] The initial homeostatic demographic regime (Stage I), in which high mortality necessitates high fertility to ensure the survival of the group, is overturned by economic and technological advances which induce a general decline in mortality rates (Stage II). The resulting high rate of natural increase precipitates the perceived need to restrain fertility at the same time that social and economic changes generate changing attitudes regarding appropriate family size and the desirability of large numbers of children (Stage III). Finally, in Stage IV, as a result of conscious efforts by parents to drastically limit the number of offspring, a new homeostasis is achieved consisting of low birth and death rates and, once again, a moderate rate of population increase. In the discussion which follows, attention will focus directly on the timing, pace, and degree of change in birth and death rates. Since theory predicts and the experience of the Petorca Valley supports the proposition that mortality change occurs prior to the fertility decline, the mortality transition will be discussed first.

Nonetheless, death rates are the most difficult of all measures to establish with any confidence, particularly from Chilean data. Mortality rates must be constructed from the combination of both births and deaths from two distinct sets of information, both of which suffer from great registration deficiencies. Nineteenth-century data for the Petorca Valley is particularly obstinate in this regard because for many decades the burial registers do not indicate parentage. Consequently, no effort could be made to link the deaths of minors in the period 1855-1884 to family histories. Moreover, infant deaths (children aged less than one year) were apparently registered very poorly indeed in the ecclesiastical records, with perhaps as many as two-thirds going unrecorded. Although deaths of children (aged one through fourteen years) are more completely recorded in the parish books, omissions for

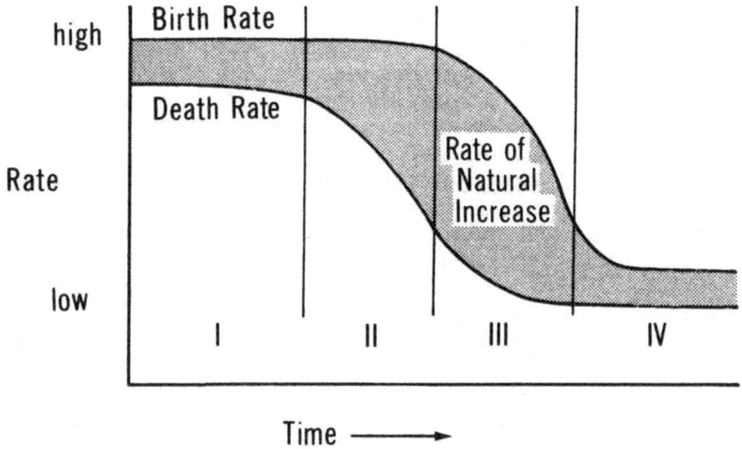

Figure 5.1 Schematic representation of the demographic transition

this age group were certainly serious until the twentieth century. Therefore, mortality rates reported here for periods prior to 1910 should be considered virtual guesses and, at the least, highly conjectural. Estimates for the twentieth century are more solidly founded and are probably highly accurate, particularly regarding the timing of change if not the actual levels of mortality.

Adult death rates do not intrude in the following discussion for two reasons. First, few writers argue the importance of changes in adult death rates for the demographic transition in general or fertility decline in particular. Most authorities contend that the impetus for restraining fertility comes from declining infant and child mortality and through the high assurance that all progeny will survive childhood. Secondly, adult mortality rates for the Petorca Valley are even more difficult to establish with certainty than those of children because of the high number of adults lacking death dates (the effects of mobility) and the wide span of years and ages to which adult deaths must be associated. Although burial registration for adults was very nearly complete after the founding of the civil registration system (1885), nonetheless their death rates are extremely difficult to calculate because of the technical difficulties in establishing the population at risk.

THE TRANSITION IN DEATH RATES

Infant and child mortality rates have been declining in the Petorca Valley for decades (Figure 5.2). Secular decline in death rates for this community may even predate by some years the founding of the local hospital (1885) or the development of a modern communication network. It would appear that for much of the nineteenth century some one-fourth of each birth cohort died during the first year of life and an additional fifth failed to survive childhood. Probably some 40 percent of each cohort died before achieving the fifteenth birthday. On the average, parents in that era had to bear five children to have three survive to adulthood. Simply turning the pages of the burial registers impresses one with the high proportion of deaths at young ages.

Wills also provide an insight into the extraordinary demographic struggles which even the richest families of the premodern era faced in trying to ensure the survival of the family lineage. The history of the Matias Cáceres clan (discussed in Chapter 2), in which only 18 of 29 children survived the father, is atypical only with regard to its exceptionally high fertility. The mortality record of the richest colonial families is remarkable for its consistency. Doña Rosa Febres, wife of one of the most important merchants in the valley at the end of the colonial era, bore thirteen children, four of whom failed to

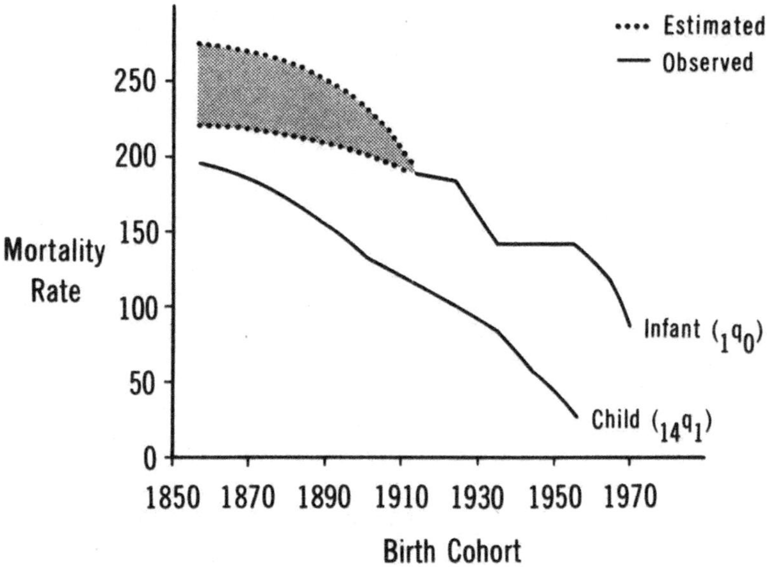

Dataset: Births (based on all infants with no restrictions)

Figure 5.2 Mortality change in the Petorca Valley

achieve majority. Don Manuel Montt, who later became president of the Republic, came from a family of seven children, three dying at very young ages.[2]

The quantitative analysis of wills in this respect, in fact, coincides closely with the burial registers (Figure 5.3). Given the very serious shortcomings in both sets of documents, the consistency of findings is remarkable. The proportion of offspring alive when parents made their wills rose very slightly from around 60 percent in the colonial epoch to a high of 65 percent at mid-nineteenth century. Afterwards, the proportion of survivors declined somewhat to about 55 percent for parents who notarized wills between 1880-1939. However, the largest and most interesting change in the whole chart occurs in the most recent period. The proportion of offspring dying before parents made their wills declined by one-half at the same time that the average age of testators rose considerably (Table 5.1).

Changing social, economic, and juridical pressures for drawing up wills makes the interpretation of small differences very difficult. Nevertheless, the two very great differences between the proportions for the two epochs (before 1930 and afterwards--referring to mortality experiences centered on a period a quarter of a century earlier) encourages one to conclude that little secular mortality decline occurred before this century.

If quibbles over the changing nature of testaments are left aside and the data are analyzed as extracted from the documents, of married testators filing in the Petorca notary and having at least one legitimate child, the mean number of dead children per family varied during earlier epochs from 2.5 to 3.7 children. For the latest group the average is only 1.2. Moreover between 80 and 90 percent of all testaments before 1930 indicate at least one dead legitimate offspring, compared with only 60 percent recently. Although serious technical problems prevent the development of refined indices showing the sole impact of mortality change on the maintenance of family lineages (see Appendix I), these data do reflect the actual experiences of an important subset of families. They demonstrate that for all premodern generations since the founding of Petorca Village the reproduction of families has been severely limited by very heavy mortality indeed. Few families raised all their offspring to maturity without at least one, and often many, dying in childhood. For earlier generations, high fertility was a demographic necessity. Without numerous progeny the vagaries of death could and did extinguish entire family lines.

SOCIETY, ECONOMY, AND THE MORTALITY DECLINE

Although wills offer an interesting perspective on the survival of legitimate heirs, a more precise picture

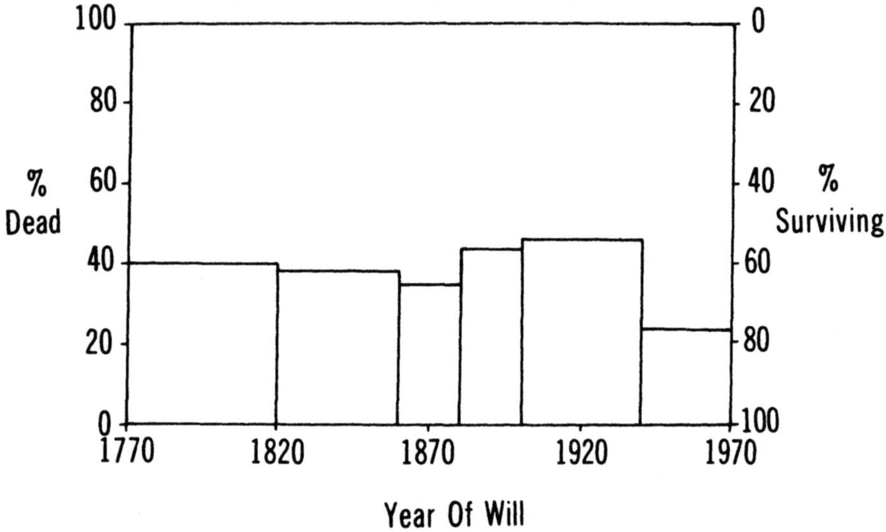

Sources and Notes: See Table 5.1

Figure 5.3 Survival of heirs as manifested in wills

TABLE 5.1
Survival of heirs: Petorca, 1770-1970

Date of Will	Number of Wills	Alive*	Dead*	Total*	Dead Offspring (%)	Testators with all Live Offspring (%)	Average Age of Testator
1770-1819	37	5.46	3.62	9.08	40.0	3	--
1820-1859	52	4.50	2.79	7.29	38.3	15	--
1860-1879	65	4.43	2.37	6.80	34.8	9	66.3
1880-1899	71	4.78	3.70	8.48	43.7	14	69.7
1900-1939	40	2.92	2.45	5.37	45.6	18	69.8
1940-1970	15	4.00	1.20	5.20	23.1	40	72.0

Sources: NP, AJP.

*Mean number of children.

NOTE: Only married (or widowed) testators aged 45 years or more with at least one legitimate offspring and survival status of each positively indicated are included here.

of the timing and magnitude of the mortality decline for infants and children in general must be constructed from the death rates (Figure 5.4). While minor fluctuations in death rates suggested by the wills cannot be elicited with any confidence from nineteenth-century burial registers, this kind of death data permits much more precision in determining the pace and scale of the mortality transition in the twentieth century. Although the quality of the estimates from the church books is very poor, a fairly substantial drop in the death rates apparently occurred before this century.

It hardly seems worthwhile to comment upon possible causes of the decline given the frailty of the data. Nevertheless it should be noted that as early as 1865 public sanitation measures and health programs became important preoccupations at all levels of government. Smallpox vaccination programs undoubtedly contributed to better health for children in particular. There were also improvements in water supplies and waste disposal. Quarantines were established rapidly whenever contagions appeared in the valley, particularly to halt the spread of smallpox and cholera. Trends in food supply and standard of living in general are more difficult to establish for lack of systematic data. Impressions gained from governors' reports and wills suggest some deterioration in the variety of diet if not in the quantity during the nineteenth century. In the late colonial period, the mineral wealth of the valley attracted a horde of petty merchants dealing in cheese, dried fish, fruits, vegetables, and the ubiquitous wines and aguardientes as well as the basics of the diet: grains and beans. By 1870 not only had this once lively commerce virtually evaporated but subsistence agriculture had deteriorated as well. Fruit trees, meticulously enumerated in estate divisions prior to 1850, gradually disappeared from the wills suggesting that orchards were no longer considered valuable or were dying out. Moreover, governors in the 1860s and 1870s noted the lack of sufficient grain even for planting as local farmers, attracted by a bourgeoning regional wheat trade, neglected supplies for their own needs. A total lack of information on gardening is unfortunate. Certainly by the middle of this century many villagers no longer planted gardens, fruit orchards were being allowed to disappear completely, and few pigs were kept in backyards (although fowl were everywhere). For several generations villagers, if not the small farmers, have become increasingly dependent upon others for their food supplies. The net effects of these developments on mortality trends simply cannot be measured.

THE TIMING AND DEGREE OF THE MORTALITY TRANSITION FOR INFANTS AND CHILDREN

If one accepts the mortality decline as depicted in

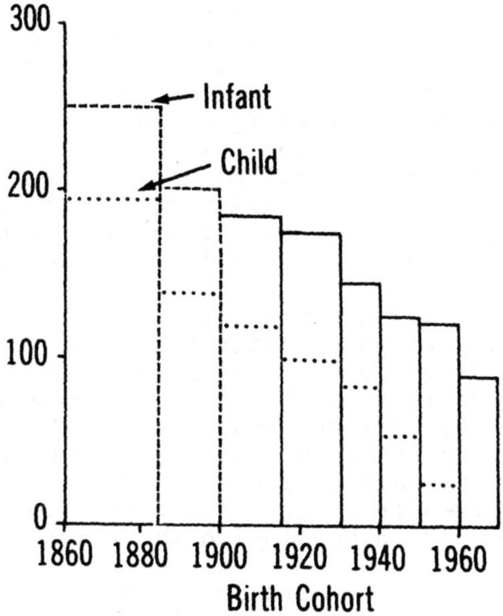

Dataset: Post 1900: At risk
Pre 1900: Births

Figure 5.4 Infant (${}_{1}q_{0}$) and child (${}_{14}q_{1}$) mortality rates: Petorca Valley, 1860-1969

Figure 5.5, death rates were still very high at the beginning of this century. The major decline in infant mortality did not occur until the Depression decade, which was followed by many years of only moderate improvements. Meanwhile, child survivalhood continued to increase substantially and steadily. The truly precipitous decline in both child and infant mortality combined must be dated from the early 1930s. Over the previous seventy years these death rates declined at an average rate of perhaps 1.0 percent per year. From 1915 through 1949 the pace increased to 1.5 percent. The most impressive relative changes occurred after 1950 when the rates declined at a rate exceeding 3.0 percent per year. Furthermore, in the early 1970s mortality decline was renewed once again. For recent years child mortality has virtually disappeared from the valley with rates lower than five deaths per thousand children (a total of eleven deaths in 1971-1976). Nevertheless, infant mortality continues to be higher than the national average; and, moreover, a slight regression appears to have begun in the last couple of years (Figure 5.5).

In general, the mortality experience of the Petorca Valley stands out in at least two respects. First, the pattern of change, both in terms of levels and pace, differs considerably from that of Chile as a whole. Petorca child mortality is lower than that of the nation, while infant death rates are higher. Secondly, the combination of rates in the valley do not correspond to any of the patterns derived from other historical populations by Coale and Demeny in developing their sets of model life tables.

The mortality transition in the Petorca Valley has been less pronounced than that for Chile. At the beginning of this century the local rates were considerably below the national figures and today they tend to equal the Chilean rates (Table 5.2). These rates do not necessarily imply that Petorca estimates are erroneous. Historically, relatively isolated rural populations have tended to show lower mortality than more densely settled regions. In an era of largely inefficacious medical technology Petorca's arid climate, sparse settlement, and geographic isolation could have blessed the community with better than average health conditions. On the other hand, when substantial doses of advanced medical technology, improvements in nutrition from rising standards of living, and developed public sanitation are required to force the death rate lower, these same characteristics work to the disadvantage of relatively impoverished rural communities like Petorca.

These considerations are particularly relevant with respect to late infant mortality (ages 1-11 months). Without well-nourished, healthy mothers and sanitary living conditions it is very difficult to decrease late infant mortality. During this century neonatal mortality (the first twenty-eight days of life) dropped by 55 percent in

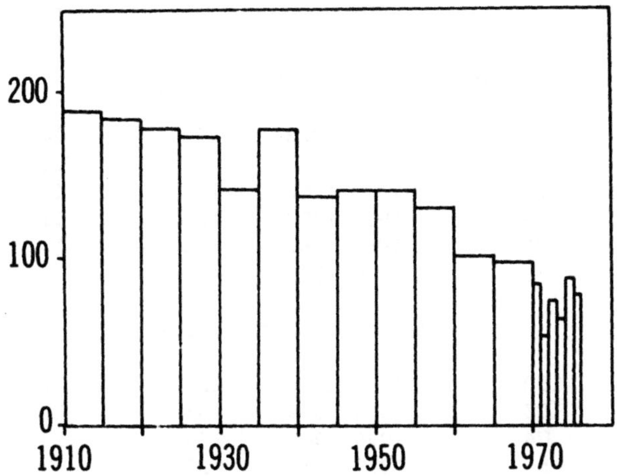

Dataset: Births. Unadjusted rates. Special tabulations for 1970-1975.

Figure 5.5 Infant mortality rates: Petorca, 1910-1975

TABLE 5.2
Infant and child mortality: Petorca Valley and Chilean rates, 1920-1960

Petorca Valley		Chile			
Birth Cohort		Period	CELADE	Arriaga	SNS
		INFANT MORTALITY RATES ($_1q_0$)			
1920-1929	176	1919-1922	250	240	
1930-1939	142	1929-1932	210	210	204
1940-1949	123	1939-1942	195	195	187
1950-1959	119	1952-1953	120	115	112
1960-1969	86	1960-1961	115	108	115
1970-1975	70	1970-1975	--	--	68
		CHILD MORTALITY RATES ($_{14}q_1$)			
1900-1914	130	1919-1922	205	240	
1915-1929	100	1929-1932	135	200	
1930-1939	84	1939-1942	130	175	
1940-1949	56	1952-1953	55	90	
1950-1959	27	1960-1961	44	55	

Datasets: At Risk (1920-1969) and Events 70 (1970-1976).

Sources: Arriaga, New Life Tables, pp. 50-64; Tacla and Somoza, "La mortalidad en Chile," pp. 271, 273; SNS, Anuario 1975 Defunciones y Causes de Muerte, p. 1.

NOTE: Petorca data refer to birth cohorts of 10 years duration while Chilean estimates are period rates.

the valley, while perinatal mortality declined at half that rate (Table 5.3). Moreover, most of the decline in perinatal death rates (1-11 months) occurred in the first stages of the mortality transition with very little improvement during the years 1950-1969. The decline for this group was 22 percent from 1930-1949 but only 7 percent for the succeeding twenty year period. Neonatal mortality, on the other hand, continued decreasing at the same pace in both periods (approximately 30 percent). Whereas neonatal mortality could be reduced with extensions of public health technology, genuine improvements in nutrition and social well being were required to ameliorate the mortality conditions for infants during the latter part of the first year of life. The economic marginality of the Petorca Valley insured that the socioeconomic transformations necessary for reducing late infant mortality

TABLE 5.3
Rate of change in infant and child mortality rates: Petorca, 1910-1975

	Infant (0-364 days)		Neonatal (0-27 days)		Perinatal (28-364 days)		Child (1-14 years)	
Birth Cohort	Rate	Δ%	Rate	Δ%	Rate	Δ%	Rate	Δ%
1910-1929	178		98		90		115	
		-26		-31		-22		-39
1930-1949	132		68		70		70	
		-22		-34		- 7		-61
1950-1969	106		45		65		27	
		-34		-40		-32		--
1970-1975	70		27		44		--	

Dataset: At Risk (1910-1969) and Events 70 (1970-1976).

would arrive tardily. Meanwhile, in the more progressive areas of Chile, both neonatal and perinatal mortality fell more rapidly from higher levels.

A further peculiarity of mortality levels in the Petorca Valley is that they do not closely approximate any of the extraordinarily complete set of stable population models developed by the Princeton University's Office of Population Research. For any given level of infant mortality in the Petorca Valley, the corresponding level of child mortality is too low when compared with the respective model life table (or vice-versa). Moreover, the tables which fit the Petorca data best are from the "East" set which no one has ever suggested as appropriate for Latin American populations.[3]

Does this incongruence mean that Petorca rates are incorrect? Probably not. The model life tables are aggregations of national experiences and therefore may not reflect the age pattern of mortality for small populations. More importantly, historical demographers have gradually recognized that there may not be any systematic relationship between infant and child mortality rates. Wrigley, in his study of Colyton (England), argued this point some years ago.[4] Moreover, the various rates of change for each age group have a certain plausibility. If mortality probabilities at specific ages are dependent upon the dynamic interaction of environmental, technological, and social forces, should we expect a golden rule of mortality in which the pattern of dying is systematically related from age group to age group and epoch to epoch?

For contemporary Petorcan families, survivalhood has become less like a game of chance in which one's possibilities are white or black, and more like a game of chess in which if one survives the first few moves, the likelihood of a premature ending becomes very small indeed. To the extent that fertility behavior is influenced by some sort of calculus for achieving a particular number of survivors, the implications of this shift are obvious. In earlier epochs, parents could realistically expect to outlive many of their children. Today the reverse is true. When infants survive the first year of life, Petorcan parents can confidently expect them to live many years, certainly well into adulthood.

TWO STAGES OF THE FERTILITY TRANSITION

The mortality transition in the Petorca Valley is associated with two major fluctuations in the fertility rate. Initially, women born during the years 1910-1924 had much higher fertility than any other cohort studied. Then, the immediately following birth cohort, 1925-1939, not only showed lower fertility, but also a larger proportion of the valley's married population began to consciously limit fertility. The fertility of the first of these cohorts can only be described with superlatives. Women born between 1910 and 1924 outdistanced the total fertility performance of previous generations by about one-half a child (9.54 versus 9.00). If the increase seems somewhat trivial, nevertheless it was sufficient to produce a noticeable rise in the overall fertility rates of the valley. Moreover, the surge in rates were intensified by an earlier age at marriage which shortened the interval between generations, accelerated the reproduction rate, and produced a greater proportion of women ultimately marrying (see Table 3.13). All these factors could account for a total increase in crude rates of two or three times the percentage observed in the total legitimate fertility rates.

The age pattern of the marital fertility increases leaves little doubt about the reality of the rising rates. They surged upward for all ages, particularly those where natality customarily falls off greatly (twenty-five through thirty-nine years; Figure 5.6). For this cohort the rates at older ages remained much higher than at any other date. On the other hand, fertility at age forty was much lower than usual.

The same configuration is observed for age at marriage specific rates (Figure 5.7). The convex shape, typical of natural fertility populations, is evident for each age at marriage as well as for the aggregated figures. Little, if any, conscious fertility control is discernible. If teenage brides show slightly lower rates beyond age twenty-five than women marrying at later ages, the differential is too slight to suggest significant birth control for this group. Moreover the fertility curve for teen brides retains its full, convex shape, the same as for women marrying at other ages.

Given the slight direct information available for investigating the causes of the upward surge in natality, any suggestions must be highly conjectural. Nevertheless,

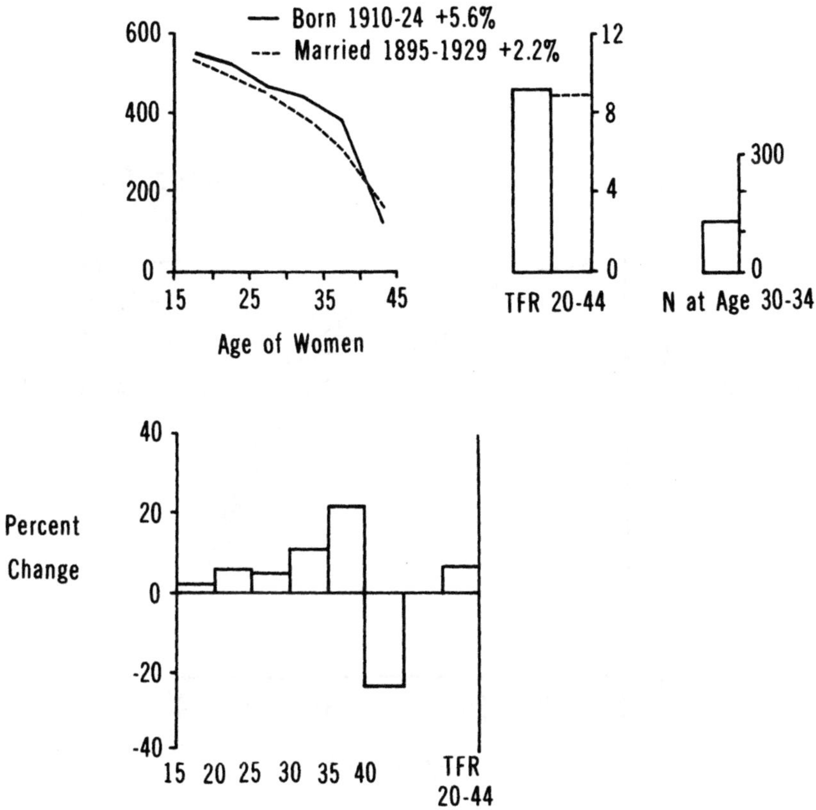

Dataset: Fertility

Figure 5.6 Fertility change for women born 1910-1924

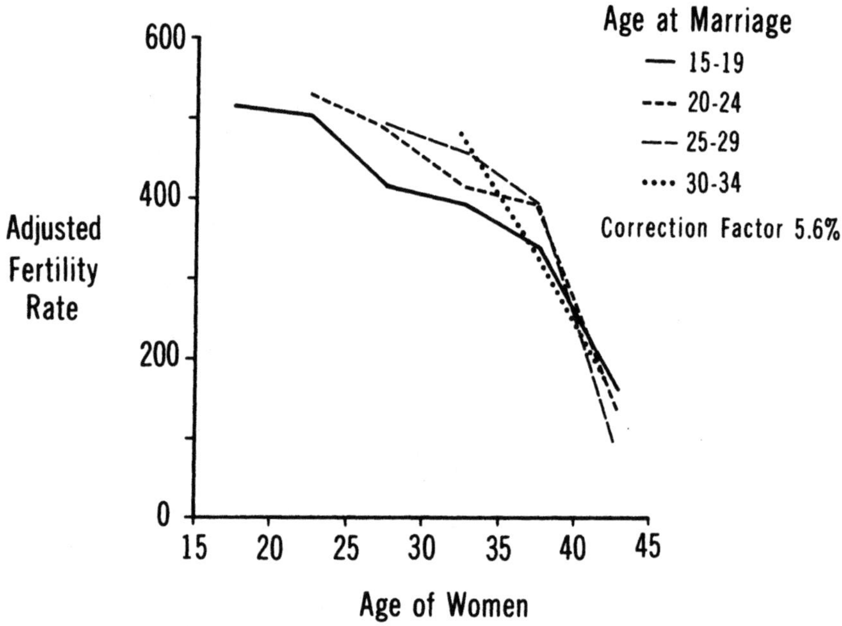

Dataset: Fertility

Figure 5.7 Fertility rates by age and age at marriage, women born 1910-1924

forces clearly operated without the conscious intervention of couples to achieve some desirable, large family size. It is very likely that this fertility increase resulted from heightened biological fecundability. In the first place, the rise occurs at all ages except the oldest. If the change resulted from a periodic event, such as an upswing in the local economy, the increase should be situated at some precise age group and related to the period in which economic conditions improved. Migration data do not imply significant economic growth. While there were no doubt ups-and-downs in the local economy, Petorcans continued to emigrate in large numbers throughout the twentieth century. The fertility trends of the poorest families also point to a biological cause. The natality rise for uneducated, illegitimate farming couples did not occur until the succeeding cohort. Apparently the conditions which forced up the fertility of most families did not have a significant impact on the poor for another fifteen years.

Support for a biological explanation also comes from the birth rates of women who were not pregnant at marriage. There is a substantial increase in the fertility for this subset in the age group at which marriage occurred. Moreover, the declining age at marriage should have produced the opposite effect: a drop because of the effects of adolescent sterility (see Figure 4.5). It seems that marital fertility rates rose because Petorcan women were physiologically capable of bearing more children rather than because they chose to bear more. With no compensatory changes in sexual behavior, coital frequency, or other social customs influencing procreation, increasing fecundability led to increased fertility.

THE CONSCIOUS CONTROL OF FERTILITY

Nonetheless, within the space of a decade or two the desire to limit one's family size became so widespread that even at the highest levels of aggregation the effects of conscious family limitation appear in the natality statistics. If the fertility of women born in the previous period must be characterized by superlatives, the experience of women born between 1925 and 1939 must be described only slightly less so (Figure 5.8). The principal differences in fertility levels between the two cohorts occur from age thirty, where the absolute and relative magnitude of the decline for the most recent cohorts is considerable. (Little attention should be given to the rates at age forty since, for the most recent cohort, they are based on very few women. Three fewer births would reduce the rate to the level of the 1910 cohort.) Moreover, this group shows an unmistakeable pattern of conscious fertility control. There is a marked, systematic differential by age at marriage. From age thirty women marrying at younger ages have lower fertility than those marrying at older

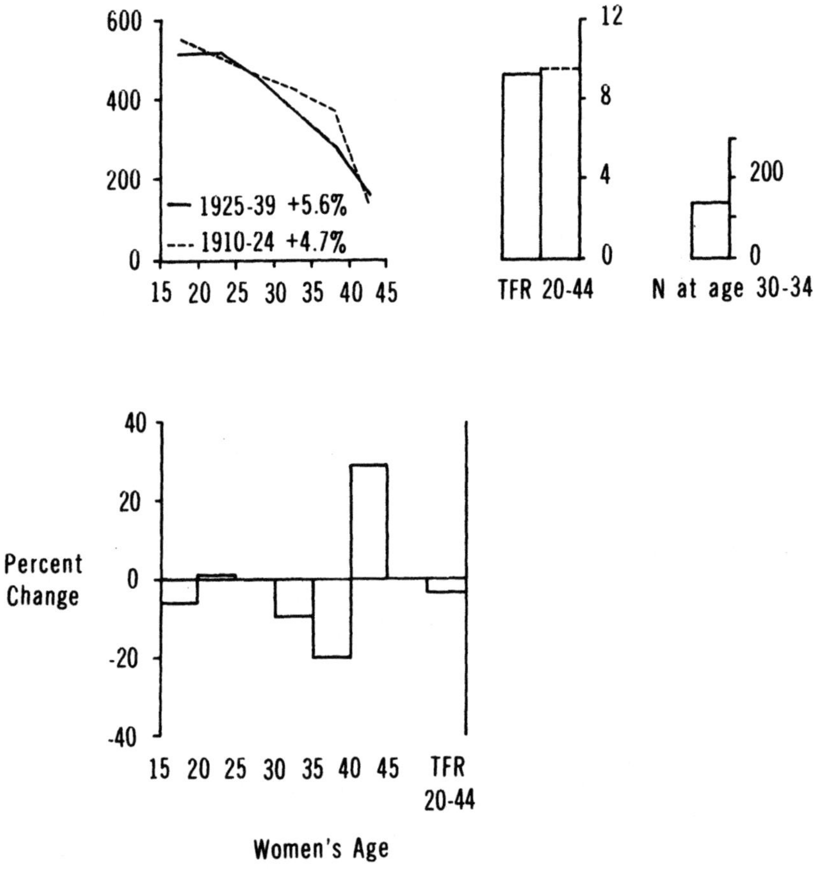

Dataset: Fertility

Figure 5.8 Fertility change for women born 1925-1939

ages. For this cohort, fertility is determined to a considerable extent by the duration of marriage. The longer a woman had been married the lower her fertility.

The contrast between the pattern of natality rates for the two cohorts by age at marriage is very marked. During the first years of marriage the most recent cohort had even higher fertility than the extraordinarily prolific one of 1910. However, within five to ten years of marriage the rates of the recent cohort were 20 percent below those of the earlier one (Figure 5.9). If the net effects of these developments were only a slight decline in the total fertility rate, the age pattern of fertility change was highly significant. For the first time in the history of the valley the aggregated figures show the unmistakeable pattern of a malthusian fertility regime: a concave curve at the older ages.

The malthusian pattern--that is, conscious fertility control once a desired family size is achieved--is even more marked for specific subsets of the population. The most impressive example is that of women not pregnant at marriage, which constituted slightly more than 40 percent of all brides in this period (versus 36.5 percent for the former; Figure 5.10). Within the space of a decade and a half total fertility for this group declined by almost 20 percent. The decline at the prime fertility limitation ages (thirty and above) were even larger, reaching 50 percent at age thirty-five. The relative significance of the transition for this group is further illustrated by comparing it with the same group of women in earlier epochs and the corresponding data for women of the same cohort with one or more premarital conceptions (Figure 5.11). Although there has always been an important difference in fertility levels by prenuptial pregnancy experience, it is only in this recent cohort that the fertility curve has become concave. The corresponding curve for all cohorts is notably convex. On the other hand, the other type of brides, those with prenuptial conceptions, continue to produce children according to natural constraints. This group had not yet begun the fertility transition.

It is interesting to note that at older ages the fertility rates for brides with no prenuptial conceptions draw closer to those of the eighteenth century Genevan Bourgeoisie rather than to those of the contemporary cohort of Petorcan women with premarital conceptions. Nonetheless, the fertility decline for this special group of Petorcan women is only partial and incomplete when compared to an historical malthusian population. Fertility rates even for the group in which the transition has already begun are 25 to 50 percent higher at ages twenty through thirty-four than for the Genevan Bourgeoisie. Moreover, poor Petorcan women of the same birth cohort (1925-1939) show the highest rates for any group in the history of the valley (Figure 5.12). Their curve is almost a flat plateau through age thirty-nine. In all

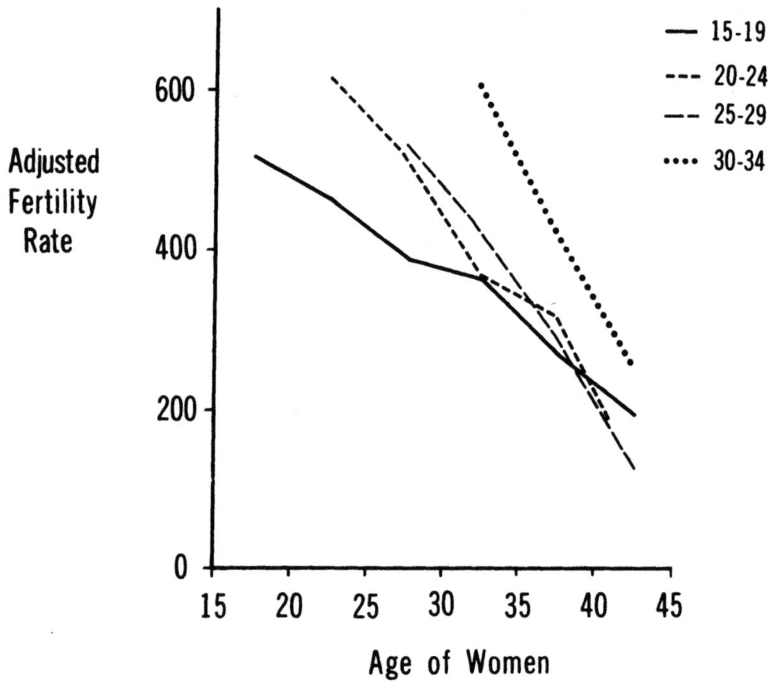

Dataset: Fertility

Figure 5.9 Fertility rates by age at marriage: women born 1925-1939

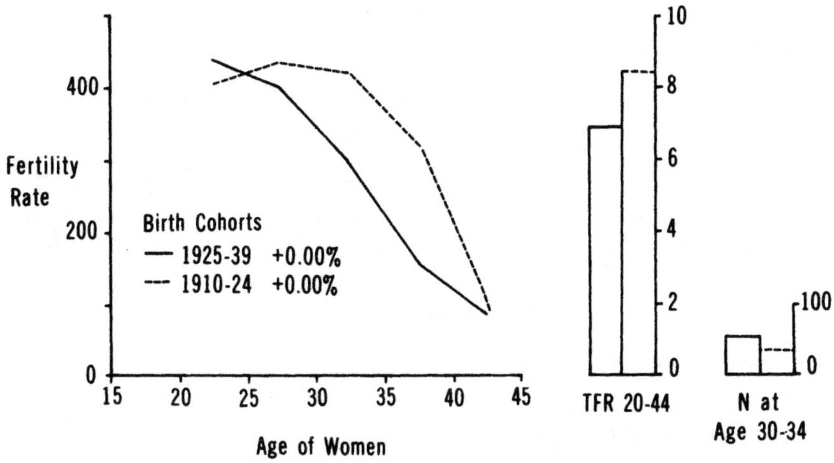

Dataset: Fertility

Note: Women excluded from age group in which marriage occurred.

Figure 5.10 Fertility transition in the Petorca Valley: subsequent natality of not pregnant brides

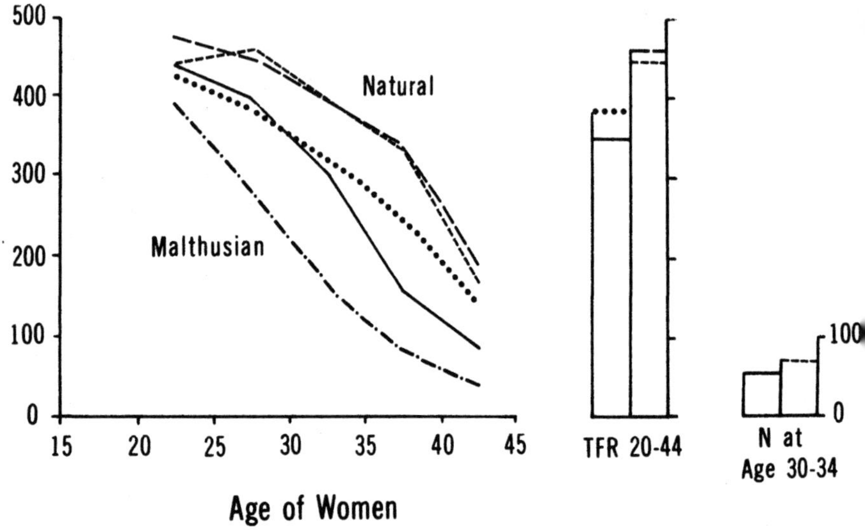

Birth Cohort, 1925-39:

— No Premarital Conceptions

--- Some Premarital Conceptions

Marriage Cohort, 1840-1969:

••• No Premarital Conceptions

—— Some Premarital Conceptions

Genevan Bourgeoisie:

·—· Husbands Born 1700-1799

Source: Fertility dataset; Henry (1956), p. 76.

Note: Women excluded from age group in which marriage occurred.

Figure 5.11 Natural and Malthusian fertility patterns

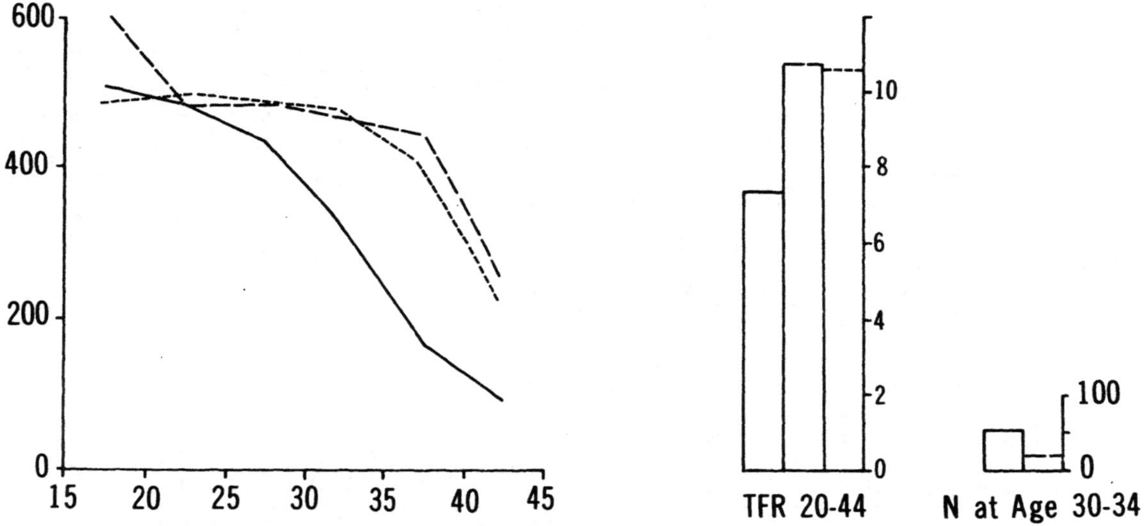

--- French Canada rates for the eighteenth century.
Petorca data refer to women born 1925-39.
—- Illiterate farmers' wives from illegitimate families.
— Brides who had no history of prenuptial conceptions.

Sources: Fertility dataset and Henripin (1954), p. 60.

Figure 5.12 Fertility patterns of two contemporary Petorcan social groups compared with an extreme natural fertility regime

essential features these women duplicated the extraordinary fertility record set by eighteenth-century French Canadians.

The reality of the fertility transition is further substantiated by both the 1970 census manuscripts for the valley and the records of the local hospital. While these data lack the historical depth of family life histories, they prove that strong differentials exist and that the trend is toward ever increasing conscious control of fertility. The census manuscripts show that, in the key ages, wives of merchants and the educated have 20 to 30 percent fewer children than farmers and the less educated (Table 5.4). There are also significant differentials according to one's residence within the valley. Women living in and around Petorca Village, the commercial and administrative center of the region, have lower fertility than those in Chincolco or nearer the <u>cordillera</u>. Even farmers' wives residing near Petorca Village have lower fertility than those located farther upstream.

Whether one is dealing with the census lists or with family histories, it is impossible to ascertain the relative importance of social or economic variables in producing the fertility transition because of the small number of cases. Moreover, the individual level data encourages one to discard single variable explanations. Legitimacy, literacy, and occupational status are all essential for creating the conditions necessary to encourage couples to limit their family size. Because of the way these attributes cluster in individual families it is impossible to statistically control for particular variables in an attempt to determine their relative importance. Moreover, on theoretical grounds one could argue that the measured variables are simply manifestations of a complex social and psychological reality which for a lack of attitudinal data must remain inscrutable to the analyst. The complexity of the premarital pregnancy variable was discussed above. Likewise, place of residence is a surrogate for the advance of medical and educational modernization in the valley. More sophisticated statistical manipulations, such as multiple classificatory analysis, prove fruitless in the effort to disentangle these relationships because of the paucity of cases, the presence of chance elements, and the way that the various attributes cluster together. The differences between subsets are too subtle and the social reality too complex to yield to more refined statistical techniques.

The demographic transition is a wholistic process and any attempt to dissect the various components, to examine first one, then another of its elements, will prove fruitless. The fertility transition in the Petorca Valley is only one aspect of the modernization process. Education, legitimization of family unions, heightened social and economic aspirations are others. On the strictly demographic side of the equation a substantial improvement in

TABLE 5.4
Mean children ever born: Petorca, 1970 census, married women

	Children Born to Women Aged 30-34	Children Born to Women Aged 35-39	Children Born to Women Aged 40-44	Number of Women Aged 30-34	Number of Women Aged 35-39	Number of Women Aged 40-44
Husband's Occupation						
Farmers (1)	5.48	6.97	6.89	27	32	19
Merchants (2)	3.86	4.41	5.25	7	17	4
Index (2/1)	70	63	76			
Women's Education						
Less than 3 years	5.19	7.35	8.00	26	31	23
3 years or more	5.17	5.38	6.47	59	55	32
Index	100	73	81			
Place of Residence						
Chincolco Upstream	5.35	6.88	7.81	54	48	37
Petorca	4.87	5.22	5.67	31	38	18
Index	91	76	73			
Farmer's Residence						
Chincolco Upstream	5.69	7.33	7.23	13	12	13
Petorca	5.29	6.75	6.17	14	20	6
Index	93	92	85			

Dataset: Pop 70.

NOTE: Women of unknown age, marital status, or fertility are excluded from the table.

life chances is not only necessary, but is assured insofar as the modernization process is a reality. In the Petorca Valley, medical technology reduced the frequency and intensity of epidemic disease and rooted out many of the endemic mortality vectors. Nevertheless, perinatal mortality remained substantial until literacy became very widespread, bastardy reduced, living standards improved, and economic prospects brightened (if only through migration elsewhere). As these developments spread up the valley, or out from Petorca Village, conscious family limitation desires and practices diffused from a narrow economic elite to an ever larger circle of the more educated, socially integrated populace.

Regarding the means by which fertility limitation was achieved, little quantitative information is available. Aside from information on induced abortions requiring medical attention, no systematic evidence for the valley exists. Withdrawal and abstention were mentioned by informants as familiar practices, but the frequency and dispersal of these methods are unknown. From the 1950s abortion data indicate a strong desire to control fertility by a noticeable portion of the valley's population. The first bit of relevant evidence extant in the hospital archives shows twenty-six women being admitted for complications following induced abortions in 1956.[5] This represented almost 8 percent of known pregnancies in the valley during that year, 10 percent of all women admitted to the hospital, and 20 percent of pregnancy-related admissions. The available serial data, which begin in 1964, show an absolute increase in abortion-related cases to thirty-seven. While the absolute number of births continued to fall (and never regained the highs of the early 1960s), complicated abortions requiring surgical intervention remained steadily in the low thirties. In 1972 when the national family planning campaign was finally extended to the valley, the discovered abortion rate was immediately reduced. Until that date folk abortions accounted for 12 to 20 percent of all pregnancy-related admissions. By 1976 the number of mal-abortions had declined by two-thirds while 95 percent of pregnant women visiting the hospital were inscribed into the family planning program. Beginning in 1974 the staff annually inserted some one hundred intrauterine devices, dispersed a slightly lower number of other contraceptive devices, performed sterilizations (17 in 1974 versus 153 deliveries), and induced a few abortions. By 1975 the number of births in the valley had declined to the lowest point since the eighteenth century. The birth rate stood at the lowest point ever. In less than ten years the crude birth rate has probably been halved, without slackening the marriage rate.[6]

The foregoing analysis is partial--many aspects of the fertility record remain unexamined--and contentious--the data are poor and the method, elaborate. Nevertheless the broad outline of the levels and patterns of childbearing is clear. Married Petorcan women in most periods and subgroups have had high natality unaffected by conscious efforts to limit family size. Only within the last generation did the values, needs, and means of family limitation become widespread. Moreover, the transition to a malthusian regime began within twenty years of a substantial, sustained decline in infant and child mortality. The process is still on-going, now extended by the dissemination of modern birth control technology. Nevertheless it is clear that a substantial decline in fertility occurred before a publicly sponsored family planning program reached the valley, that is, without the widespread use of contraceptives.

As this study concluded, neither the mortality nor fertility transition had terminated. In the classic four stage paradigm of the demographic transition, Petorcans are still in Stage III with birth rates falling fast and death rates more slowly. It is unclear how soon or at what levels a new homeostasis will be achieved.

NOTES

1. Beaver, Demographic Transition Theory, pp. 33-40.

2. NP, Vol. 4, f. 197; vol. 8, f. 25, 161.

3. Ansley J. Coale and Paul Demeny, Regional Model Life Tables and Stable Populations (Princeton, N.J., 1966), pp. 442-445.

4. E. A. Wrigley, "Mortality in Pre-Industrial England: The Example of Colyton, Devon, Over Three Centuries," Daedelus, Vol. 97, p. 570, ff. After the final typescript was prepared further corroboration for this argument came to my attention: John Knodel and Hallie Kinter, "The Impact of Breast Feeding Patterns on the Biometric Analysis of Infant Mortality," Demography, Vol. 14 (1977), pp. 406-407.

5. Informe Anual 1956, Centro de Salud de Petorca, 12.

6. Data graciously provided to me by the Petorca Hospital Statistician, Srta. Adriana González.

6
Petorca and the Population History of Chile

Within the span of a single generation the people of the Petorca Valley experienced a profound transformation in marriage behavior, life expectancy, and fertility patterns. The purpose of this chapter is to relate these demographic changes to an explanatory paradigm, and to compare the pace and degree of local changes with national tendencies.

POPULATION TRANSITIONS AND MODERNIZATION

The modernization paradigm explains the principal secular demographic and social changes in the Petorca Valley. Contemporary academic fashions justifiably dictate that one deal with modernization theory cautiously. Nevertheless, the concept has linguistic and analytical superiority over competing explanatory paradigms, principally because even the most perceptive critics are unable to present any alternative.[1] If the vagueness of modernization theory dulls the senses, if its ethnocentric roots arouse passions, still, some concept is required to express the social, demographic, and attitudinal discontinuities inherent in the extraordinary changes occurring in the Third World in this century. Abolish the word, but the concept remains. Moreover, the word "modernization" is more than linguistic opportunism or the shorthand of a cynical scholar.[2] Modernization theory directs attention to pertinent structures, processes, and analytical categories. For understanding the process of demographic change and innovation at the community level (as opposed to that of nations or the world), the concept may be particularly useful.

Given the narrow focus of this study I have no interest in attempting to elaborate a general theory of modernization. Rather, for the present purposes, the argument narrows to two specific points which are shared by most elaborations of the modernization idea. In the first place, modernization means a dramatic transition in behavior, in this case mainly demographic and social. In the preceding discussion this has been explicitly recognized by the use of the phrase "demographic transition." Secondly, the transition is a multifaceted, integral process.[3] Rates of change of various social and economic phenomena are interrelated--growth of industry with expansion of wage labor, spread of mass education with increasing power of the state bureaucracy, mortality decline with rising standards of living--but in a complex and necessarily variable fashion from region to region and nation to nation. Because of the very complexities by which these factors and others interact, the paths toward modernization are varied indeed with regard to specific relationships between indicators. Notwithstanding the systemic nature of transformations, modernization does not necessarily mean economic, technological, or cultural convergence. Both critics and perceptive supporters alike note that repetition of the European historical experiences is impossible (and undesirable). There is a wide variety of patterns in terms of degree, timing, and pace of change. Finally, the process is an open-ended one, not a state--just as in other analytical traditions imperialism, under-development, or primitive accumulation are considered processes.[4]

With regard to population change, it is apparent that the demographic transition paradigm is a generalization about which there is considerable variability when specific historical cases are studied. In some European regions fertility change preceded economic growth; in others, malthusian patterns apparently became firmly established before economic or mortality change had gone very far. Nevertheless, demographic, economic, and social change have tended to be related, although not directly nor in a simple linear fashion. Wherever its occurrence the process is complex, uneven, and always unfinished.

The demographic transition paradigm correctly directs attention to mortality decline and the conscious control of fertility. The fashionable disgust and premature burial of the demographic transition concept (". . . it neither said nor explained anything . . . ."[5]) is certainly unwarranted with respect to Chilean history in general or that of the Petorca Valley in particular. The conscious control of family size without the motivation of subsistence crisis, falling income, or political coercion, is certainly a momentous social and psychological transformation.

In broad outline the stages of population change in the Petorca Valley correspond to the stages of the demographic transition paradigm. While infant and child mortality rates have declined for many decades, the rates of change increased greatly during two periods of this century (1930-1950 and 1960-1973). In recent years even the age group most resistant to improvements, infants aged 1-11 months, has yielded to the efforts of parents and health workers. Although considerable improvement in survivalhood occurred by 1930, nevertheless, even at that late date perhaps 30 percent of each generation died before attaining adulthood. In recent years the proportion has dropped to about 10 percent. Now parents are not only assured of surviving heirs, but of virtually all offspring achieving adulthood once the first year of life has been attained. To the extent that parents ever speculate about their children's survival chances, today they may realistically hope to achieve even their highest expectations.

Aggregated fertility data for Petorca imply that expectations have been very high indeed. An analysis of the histories grouped into broad periods shows a slow rise in marital fertility at most ages, even for the most recent cohort. However, as early as the 1950s, a large subgroup of the population began to moderately limit family size. Natality differentials for earlier periods seem to be less the result of conscious control than of socially related inhibitions.

In the Petorca Valley mortality decline preceded family limitation which only began on a large scale once infant mortality levels had dropped by some two-thirds. The earliest conscious birth control was detected for the more educated population living near the hospital. Meanwhile, a second subset of the same cohort achieved levels almost identical to those of the exceptionally fecund French Canadians of the eighteenth century. Shortly, fertility control spread very rapidly to women of all social backgrounds, according to aggregate data for the 1970s. Within two decades of rapid mortality decline family limitation had become established (1950-1960). Within another decade (1965-1975), birth control had become omnipresent. The transition from virtually no conscious birth control to almost total control took less than twenty-five years. This change in behavior does not mean that the demographic experience of Petorcans approaches those of contemporary Europeans; however, it is closer to European levels than Petorcan ones at the beginning of this century. Nevertheless, both Petorcan infant mortality and marital fertility remain at least as twice as high as European levels.

The mortality transition was also accompanied by a marriage transition. By 1920 Petorcans began to marry in greater proportions and at younger ages than in previous generations. When a new plateau had been achieved (1940), the median age at first marriage for women had declined by almost three and one-half years (Table A4.2). While family formation is usually ignored in discussion of the demographic transition, changing marriage patterns have clearly been very significant in the Petorca Valley. The marital structure of the settled population has been transformed. A vastly greater proportion of women now become heads of stable family unions at younger ages (Table 3.13) and, with lower adult mortality rates, most remain family heads throughout the fecund years.

The three main components of population reproduction--

marriage, mortality, and fertility--have all reinforced each other in accelerating the potential rate of natural increase in the valley. Although the greatest impact on population growth came from the declining death rate (principally infant and child mortality), marriage and fertility changes have been important as well. (Crude rates are not presented for the valley because changing population structure of small communities robs simple demographic measures of their substantive value. One of the curious ironies of family reconstitution is that complex cohort measures are perfectly feasible but simple point estimates are not.) Earlier and more widespread marriage should have added one or two additional children to total family size with rising fertility rates contributing perhaps an additional half. That the total population of the valley stagnated indicates that a surge of out-migration largely offset effects of the disequilibrium associated with stage two of the transition. Initially, this was the principal demographic response to mortality decline. Most other nondemographic responses may be significant but are not quantifiable nor are the relations direct. For example, leftist political parties began to attract support for the first time in the 1930s. Voting results from earlier decades are monotonously uniform with virtually all votes going to a single party or candidate. In the 1938 election the Popular Front presidential candidate polled 40 percent of the vote in the valley.[6]

The facts of population change seem clear; the explanation is more obscure. Data--serial, sporadic, or otherwise--for key elements of the modernization equation do not exist: local capital flows, occupational histories, income per head, desired family size, life style expectations, etc. At this point it is necessary to go beyond what has been elicited from the demographic data to place the population trends of the valley within a more wholistic framework, even if much of the discussion boils down to nothing more than deductive theorizing. Attention is focused on the most perplexing aspect of the transition: fertility decline.

The linkages between fertility change and modernization are both attitudinal and structural. For Petorcans the perception of their circumstances and opportunities must have been as important as their conjunctural realities. Clearly the amount of strictly economic development which has taken place in the valley is very small indeed. Beginning early in this century the public service sector--the hospital staff, schoolteachers, police, and government administrators--expanded in size and public salaries became more regular and competitive. Nevertheless, primary or secondary activities--farming, mining, and commerce--hardly expanded at all; quite the contrary, their economic viability became increasingly precarious. The local economy became ever more dependent upon the outside as Petorcan enterprises failed to weather the competitive storm generated by the transportation revolution. As long as goods everywhere were transported by pack-mule and ox-cart, the Petorca economy was competitive. Once the railroad and steamship arrived in Chile, the valley's geographic isolation sheltered local artisans, shopkeepers, farmers, and ranchers who maintained a certain prosperity by producing for, selling to, and servicing the local microeconomy. After the railroad penetrated the valley, independent production suffered severely. Not even the local baker could compete. Finally in 1953, after sixty years of publication, the village newspaper, Voz de Petorca, shut down; while increasing literacy expanded its potential readership five-fold, Santiago newspapers were as cheap and more desirable.

Petorcans who remained in the valley underwent a process of pauperization. The townspeople were forced into petty commerce, hawking food and small articles from the front door or letting rooms.[7] At the beginning of this century the number of licenses for petty commerce jumped several fold. Detailed occupational histories are unavailable but it is clear that the decline of the local economy forced both men and women to scrounge as never before at the same time that Petorcans fled in search of opportunities elsewhere. There were no subsistence crises nor widespread, effective efforts to change economic structures. At the end of the colonial era, Petorca was probably one of the richest rural communities in the Captaincy-General of Chile. For later times income figures are not available, but today the public health authorities consider Petorca as the poorest in its region; family income is probably several times below the national average. According to official hospital estimates, in 1976, 34 percent of preschool children suffered from "undernourishment" (up from 24 percent in 1975).[8] Therefore, direct economic inducements of the type that figure most prominently as explanations of fertility change at the macrolevel have little relevance for the situation in the Petorca Valley. Rather, the most important linkages are social change, mortality decline, and change in attitudes.

If national economic development generated pauperism and local underdevelopment, nevertheless there has been significant social development. The most important element must be the sharp decline in illiteracy which occurred in two stages: 1880-1900 and 1925-present (Table 6.1). The growth of literacy and the penetration of this isolated community by the mass media increased the quantity and range of available information. In earlier epochs, communication was principally oral. Awareness of new modes of behavior came through personal experience, chatting with acquaintances and relatives, or listening to the orders of a priest, mine owner, or farm administrator. Literacy liberated Petorcans from parochial informants and made available more cosmopolitan and varied information about their social, economic, and political conditions (if

TABLE 6.1
Ability to sign name by bride's birth cohort: Petorca Valley, 1820-1954

Bride's Birth Cohort	Bride and Groom Signed (percentage)	Both Marked "X" (percentage)	Number of Cases
1820-1839	4.5	83.6	1076
1840-1859	10.2	76.9	974
1860-1879	16.3	60.8	887
1880-1894	31.3	36.0	400
1895-1909	38.7	22.3	488
1910-1924	47.5	17.6	488
1925-1939	66.8	9.7	506
1940-1954	72.8	7.0	272

Dataset: Marriage.

NOTE: The substantial rise for the 1880 cohort is the result of education advances, relatively greater acceptance of civil marriage by the literate population and the exclusion of Hierro data from consideration. The 1940-1954 cohort is incomplete; the literacy ratio will increase as the cohort completes its marriage history.

only to a limited degree). The completion of the rail link, and much later the introduction of regular bus service, increased contacts between resident Petorcans and relatives, friends, and workmates who had migrated to Santiago, Valparaíso, and nearby towns. Cheap, rapid transport was particularly important for women, whose travel had been restricted to the slow-gaited mule or walking. The development of mass media and mass transportation unquestionably influenced mentalities with regard to economic expectations, life style, family customs, and ultimately family size.

New ideas about work, family, and life style spread through the valley, even though in many cases local economic realities seriously contradicted expectations. With regard to birth control, in the initial stages the most important content of the innovative attitudes was not technique, but rather the idea that there were alternatives to the customary pattern of childbearing where physiological conditions and social norms determined the number of offspring. The key element was a desire to manipulate family size according to one's wishes. This attitude was entangled within the same bundle that brought information about new economic and social opportunities.

The pattern of diffusion of birth control ideas was not strictly class defined; however, while communication across class lines was obviously commonplace, intrafamily information flows were most important for changing fertility behavior. Contacts between friends and family who had migrated to the city were probably decisive in this respect. Only in the 1970s with the initiation of a strong birth control program did interclass diffusion (or coercion) become significant for changing the fertility behavior of Petorcans.

The better educated, more accommodated parents consciously restricted their fertility at an earlier date because of their receptivity to new ideas and behavior. This group was propitiously placed to pluck the fruits of social and economic change as the valley was planted with ever-extravagant symbols of a better tomorrow. It is not without significance that the largest group showing the earliest and sharpest conscious restraints on fertility included precisely those couples who complied earliest with the vital registration laws. Those who from the start recognized, sought, or simply accepted the benefits of a legally constituted family were precisely those who first responded to the rewards for restraining natural procreation. They adopted birth control measures on their own before the government family planning campaign penetrated the valley and before modern contraceptive methods became available there. Their choice appears to have been totally voluntary and self motivated.

However, for less educated parents with fewer means and perhaps less hope for social or economic mobility, family limitation involved more direct coercion, enticement, or persuasion. After a formal campaign was initiated in 1972 a highly motivated staff sought to counsel every woman entering the local hospital about family planning opportunities and supply her with contraceptives if desired. For this group of women conscious fertility control accompanied rather than preceded behavioral or attitudinal changes with regard to socioeconomic circumstances. This was clearly an interclass facilitated innovation, if one considers the hospital professionals as middle class. Notwithstanding the use of formal counseling and free contraceptives to encourage the less educated women to limit their fertility, this was an opportune juncture between the desires of women using the hospital and the plans of the public health service. An extraordinary, immediate drop in fertility was registered with the introduction of technical contraceptive methods. Neither premiums nor monetary inducements of any kind were used as an enticement. The hospital staff was also sensitive to questions of individual liberty and choice. While the difference between education and coercion can become obscure when an enthusiastic public servant embarks upon a crusade, in this instance, the coercive aspects of the program were minimal.

The speed with which conscious family limitation became the accepted norm is most impressive. There are no firm indications of widespread birth control in the Petorca

Valley prior to 1950. Most of the family limitation measured in the pedigrees occurred in the 1960s. Within fifteen years the process had spread throughout the valley.

THE DEMOGRAPHIC TRANSITION IN CHILE

If attitudes and aspirations provided motivation for the initial spread of family limitation, mortality decline established the essential demographic context for all types of families, those with premarital births as well as those without. Apparently, in European demographic history the relationship between mortality and fertility change has not been systematic. In Chile, however, mortality decline appears to have been a sufficient cause for malthusian fertility patterns to emerge and very rapidly predominate. Nevertheless, mortality decline was accompanied by both social development and real economic growth in a dynamic national economy.

The Chilean demographic transition probably began at the turn of the century, but a sharp decline in mortality dates from 1936 (Figure 6.1). There were three phases in the mortality decline. During phase one (1936-1956) infant mortality declined by 50 percent from 225 deaths per thousand live births to 108, an average annual decline of 2.5 percent. During the following decade neonatal mortality (0-28 days) hardly declined at all and severely retarded the overall rate of change. In 1967 the downward trend was renewed. By 1975 the infant mortality rates stood at 55, less than one-fourth the level of half a century earlier. Petorca departed from a much lower mortality level than the Chilean national rate (180 versus 240 in 1920), declined more slowly, and gradually moved above the national average. In 1975 the Chilean infant mortality rate stood at 55 versus 75 for the Petorca Valley and 43 for Santiago province.[9]

The timing and pace of national fertility change are more obscure because of inadequately published data. The vital statistics data are unsuitable until 1952 and after that date regional estimates may be made only for census years. Moreover the 1970 vital data are not yet available. Finally, the national and regional figures are cross-sectional rates while the Petorca figures are cohort experiences. The Petorca rates for the most recent cohort are considerably above the national figures except at age thirty-five and beyond for Petorca women who had no premarital conceptions (Figure 6.2). Petorca rates are much more convex while the national figures have a gentle almost rectilinear slope. Relative to 1953, the Chilean rates for 1960 show a general increase at all ages. After that short-lived surge, marital fertility fell dramatically. The national figures for 1966 deviate sharply from earlier patterns; the pronounced concave gradient beginning at age twenty-five indicates very substantial conscious

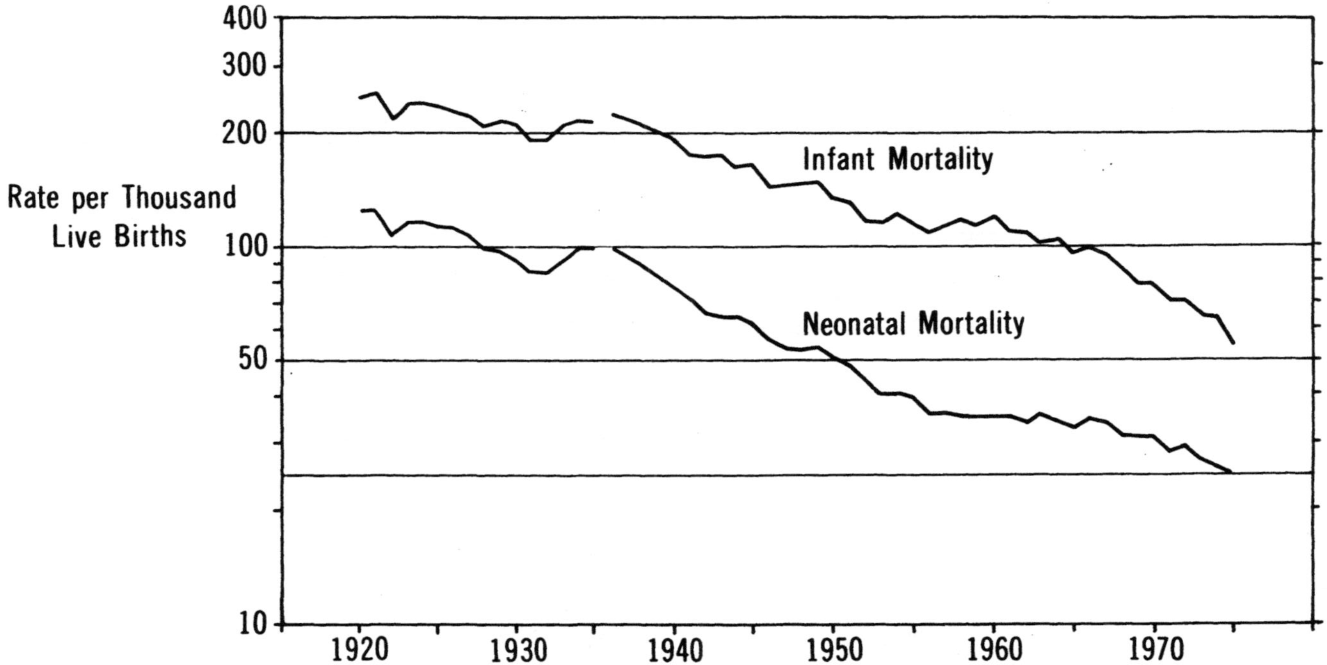

Sources: INE (1953), xv (for 1920-1935); SNS (1975a), 1 (for 1936-1975).
Semi-logarithmic scale.

Figure 6.1 Infant and neonatal mortality trends: Chile, 1920-1975

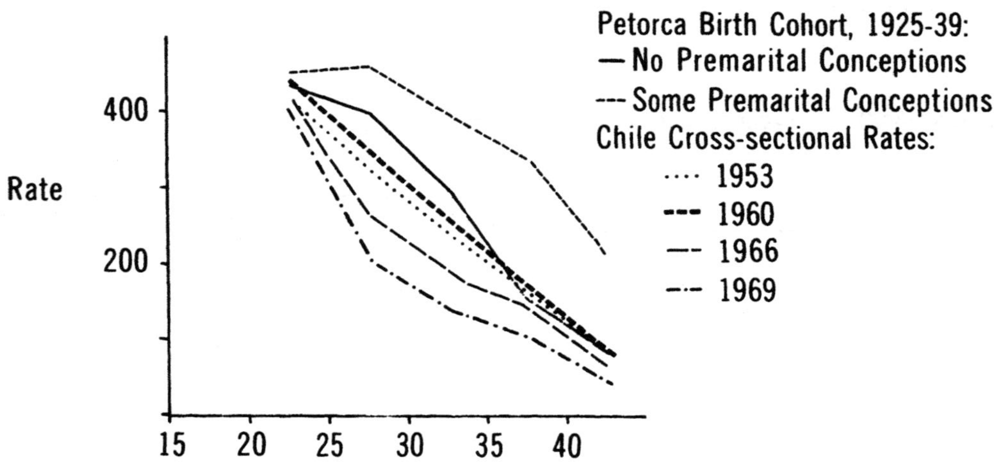

Sources: Fertility dataset. INE (1953), 17; (1960b), 15; (1966), 3, 43; United Nations (1975), 768. 1960 rates recalculated with married women from census: INE (1960a), Table 5A.

Note: Women are excluded from age group in which marriage occurred.

Figure 6.2 Marital fertility after midtwentieth century Chile and Petorca

TABLE 6.2
Crude birth rates for selected provinces, 1953-1975 (births per thousand inhabitants)

	1953	1960	1975
Aconcagua	34	40	23
Santiago	35	34	23
Colchagua	38	39	25
Chile	35	36	25

Sources: INE (1953), pp. 7, 8; (1960b), pp. 5-7; (1960a), Table 1; SNS (1975), p. 2.

family limitation. By 1969 rates had dropped enormously. At age twenty-five and above marital fertility levels had declined by almost 50 percent in only nine years.

Regional patterns of marital fertility in 1960 were diverse (Figure 6.3). Santiago already showed a slight concave pattern at that date and stood some 25 percent below the rates for rural provinces, such as Colchagua and Aconcagua. The pattern for Aconcagua province very closely approximated that of Petorca women without premarital conceptions, while Colchagua rates were considerably higher, more convex, and similar to Petorca women who had premarital conceptions. Incipient fertility control was already notable at the provincial level in the case of Aconcagua, but Colchagua at that date was characterized by a natural fertility regime. Marital fertility data are not presently available for 1970, but the crude birth rates give some general indications of the drastic fertility changes which have occurred recently (Table 6.2). The national rate rose slightly from 1953 to 1960 because declining fertility at older ages was insufficient to offset both increased proportions of married women at fertile ages (principally the result of declining spinsterhood) and the upward surge in marital fertility below age forty. While many factors influenced the actual level of the crude rates in 1975, most of the decline was the result of family limitation and the government assisted birth prevention program. The decline occurred in rural provinces like Colchagua as well as urban ones. Within fifteen years, modern fertility patterns had spread throughout much of the Chilean countryside. High fertility remained only in the far south.

The pattern of demographic change in the Petorca Valley and Chile as a whole suggests that there is a marked interrelationship between marriage, fertility, mortality, and both socioeconomic realities and aspirations. The

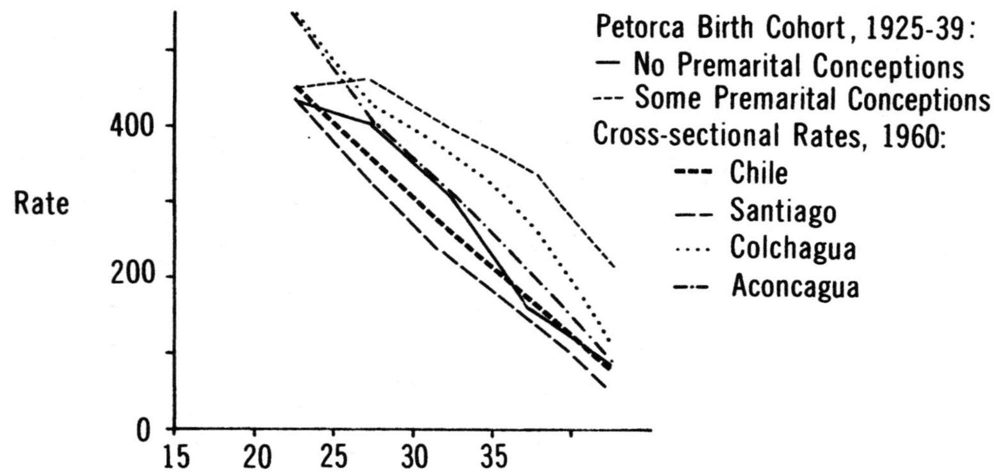

Sources and Notes: See Figure 6.2

Figure 6.3 Marital fertility 1960: Chile, three provinces, and Petorca

incredibly rapid fertility decline in Chile was made possible by a very substantial decline in mortality and the dissemination of a birth control program in response to considerable demand for these services in both the cities and the countryside.

If a modern demographic regime reigns in the Petorca Valley it is without the economic and social trappings which characterized European communities at a similar demographic stage. Chilean experience shows how far a country may go in achieving a modern demographic structure without escaping the bonds of dependency, underdevelopment, and social inequality. The recent chaos and violence is only the most dramatic manifestation of the costly, difficult struggle waged by the Chilean people. It is unclear whether modern population patterns will help or hinder them in their struggle for social dignity, political equality, cultural autonomy, and economic independence.

NOTES

1. See Dean C. Tipps, "Modernization Theory and the Comparative Study of Societies: A Critical Perspective," Comparative Studies of Society and History, Vol. 15 (1973), pp. 199-226, for a thorough critique. Raymond Grew, "Modernization and Its Discontents," American Behavioral Scientist, Vol. 21 (1977), pp. 289-312, surveys the literature for the historian.

2. E. A. Wrigley, "The Process of Modernization and the Industrial Revolution in England," Journal of Interdisciplinary History, Vol. 3 (1972), pp. 225-259.

3. Oechsli and Kirk, "Modernization and the."

4. Martha E. Giminez recently elaborated a theoretical paradigm for analyzing Latin American Population dynamics in which imperialism is the key element: "Population and Capitalism," Latin American Perspectives, Vol. 4 (1977), pp. 5-40.

5. D. E. C. Eversley, "Review of Population Patterns in the Past," Demography, Vol. 14 (1977), p. 546.

6. Mr. Paul Drake kindly collected voting statistics for the Petorca Valley from a variety of official sources.

7. Lenin developed a prescient theoretical explanation for the growth of pauperism and underemployment "on the [economic and geographic] regional frontiers of capitalism." See B. Ia. Smulevich, Críticas de las teorías y la política burgesas de la población (Santiago, 1971), p. 20.

8. Reported by the hospital statistician, Andriana González.

9. Servicio Nacional de Salud, Anuario 1975 Defunciones y causas de muerte (Santiago, 1976), p. 2; and Nacimientos (Santiago, 1976), p. 1. Petorca data from local civil registries.

APPENDIX I
Critique of Demographic Registers

The assessment of error and bias is an important consideration in the analysis of family life histories. The widely discussed deficiencies of the Chilean vital events records immediately prejudice conclusions derived from them, and the lack of any historical studies to provide methodological guidelines for the successful exploitation of these highly suspect documents should arouse a skeptical curiosity about the competence with which the project has been carried out. Consequently, questions about data quality and methods of elaboration are particularly important. The quality of family histories and the confidence in the demographic measures elicited from them depend upon three closely intertwined problems: the representativeness of the reconstitutable families, biases in the reported data and the method of elaboration, and omission of events from the registers.

If an extraordinarily presumptuous leap of faith and rather careful reasoning is required to project the demographic tendencies discovered in Petorca to all of Chile, is it even likely that the reconstructed family histories are representative of the life experiences of all the people who lived in the valley? The description of the procedure followed to build the histories indicates that very little information is available for many families. People moved into the community, stayed a short while and moved on without a trace in the official records. Some transients fell ill and died in the community leaving a few small, but for research purposes virtually useless, facts about their lives. Fairly elaborate information about each individual and each family is required to contribute to the examination of basic changes in mortality and fertility. The date of marriage of the parents is essential for all except the most rudimentary social analysis. Only full histories with birth, death, and marriage dates of the husband and wife can be exhaustively analyzed and form the basis for much of the strictly demographic analysis.

TABLE A1.1
Distribution of children appearing in vital registers of study area by birth period and legitimacy

	Children of Parents Married in Area				
Period of Birth	Born After Marriage (%)	Born Before Marriage (%)	Natural Children (%)	Legitimate, Parents Married Elsewhere (%)	Total
1840-1864	49.4	9.1	20.0	21.5	10,880
1865-1884	46.8	10.4	26.6	16.2	6,739
1885-1914	44.5	12.0	26.3	17.2	8,993
1915-1929	40.4	20.8	26.4	12.4	3,086
1930-1939	46.3	17.0	19.6	17.1	2,540
1940-1949	50.5	14.1	16.8	18.5	2,595
1950-1959	49.3	13.4	15.1	22.2	2,806
1960-1964	49.4	8.8	15.4	26.4	1,408
1965-1970	50.2	5.7	18.9	25.1	1,409
Total					40,456

Dataset: Births.

REGISTRATION PRACTICES AND METHODOLOGICAL IMPLICATIONS

The distribution of children according to the marital status of their parents (Table A1.1) illustrates the implications of changing social and administrative realities for the interpretation of the demographic rates derived from this study. Proportionately fewer children were born before marriage during the period 1885-1914 than during any other period prior to 1960. The sharp increase observed in the proportion of children born before civil marriage from 1915 through 1929 reflects the hesitancy that many parents had about the importance of the newly mandated civil ceremonies. Later, as religious objections wore away and the social and legal benefits of civil marriage increased, fewer Petorcans were born prior to their parents' civil union. The technical ramifications of the ebb and flow of people's compliance with the legal registration procedures are substantial. For example, in analyzing changing family formation patterns based on observed birth intervals within marriage, from 6 to 20 percent of the children must be excluded because they were born prior to the legal union of the family. The Table indicates that an additional 12 to 25 percent are lost because their parents married before migrating into and bearing children in the community. After illegitimate children are excluded, only 40 to 50 percent of all children remain in the analysis. The criteria for the inclusion of families becomes even more restrictive in deriving other estimates, such as age-specific fertility rates where families lacking the death date of the first-dying spouse must be rejected. These analyzable subsets only hazily mirror the experience of the valley's inhabitants. Families which drifted in and out of the records, whether by migration or by haphazard compliance with registration laws, probably differed substantially from their civilly responsible, sedentary neighbors. Extremely selective inclusion criteria--which may be necessary to control for intervening variables, increase the reliability of the data, or meet the requirements for calculating particular rates--sharply reduce the number of families. Nevertheless, substantial advances in demographic history have been made through the analysis of a remarkably small proportion of reconstituted families. Etienne Gautier and Louis Henry, on the basis of only 118 life histories of the villagers of Crulai, argued that as late as the mid-eighteenth century the community constituted a preMalthusian population practicing no discernible fertility control. Those histories comprised less than 20 percent of the births and marriages inscribed in the Crulai parish records during the period 1674-1742.[1] There are at least two essential ingredients in the successful projection of a relationship derived from a small subset of reconstituted families on the larger, target population: analysis of the relevant sociodemographic differences between the included and the excluded families, and the elaboration through a process of historical, demographic, and statistical reasoning of the implications of the divergencies for the argument.

Throughout this study tests of statistical significance have not been applied to any quantitative results. These statistics have been omitted for two reasons. In the first place demographic historians customarily shun these techniques, whether from ignorance, choice, or utter exhaustion. Secondly, I chose not to apply them here because they are methodologically inappropriate and statistically weak. The data are not drawn from a sample. Quite the contrary, the material used here consists of all the data which can be assembled about the sometime inhabitants of the valley. When subsets of these histories are selected to study particular problems and comply with specific rules, it is with a clear recognition that the subsets are not scientific samples but rather clumps of data analyzable according to explicit systematic rules. Tests of significance in such circumstances hinder rather than promote understanding. With regard to the possibility of using such tests to estimate the effects of random error, they are too weak to provide guidelines when one recognizes that the principal components of error and bias are both substantial and nonrandom. Throughout, the emphasis is upon major differences rather than minor ones. In these circumstances statistical tests may serve a psychological function but they do not serve to elucidate relationships.[2]

While the problem of representative data plagues all reconstitution studies, there are three biases peculiar to this study: the method used to link illegitimate children into families, the determination of children's birth ranks, and the effects of abruptly terminating the histories in 1970.

LINKING ILLEGITIMATE CHILDREN

Given the prevalence of bastards in this community (more elegantly referred to as natural children in Spanish), it is important to correctly link them to their corresponding mothers. Matching problems arise because with only one parent given, it is sometimes difficult to determine whether two infants belong to the same or two different mothers. In sorting out the children of mothers with common names, the mothers' Christian names, place of residence, and age and witness information were used. Where there was a close correspondence in the mother's birthdate and a match on all names and place of residence, links could be made with some certainty. At other times, confident links were made because a grandmother or uncle repeatedly acted as a witness to the inscriptions. Table A1.2 demonstrates some matching difficulties and their resolutions.

Initially all infants born to mothers with the same

TABLE A1.2
Linking ambiguities: natural children lacking father's family name (mothers with the most common Christian and family names, 1831-1958)

Family Number	Mother's Christian Name	Children's Birthdates	Children's Birthplace	Mother's Birthdate	Mother's 2nd Family Name*	Witness
1	Maria Nieves	1831,33,35	"Petorca"	--	--	--
2	Maria	1840,41,43, (1845,1848)	Hierro Viejo (Church)	--	--	--
3	Maria	1849	Out of valley	--	--	--
4	Maria	1860,69,70	Chincolco	--	--	--
5	Maria	1875	Out of valley	--	--	--
6	Maria	1897	Chincolco	1861	--	--
7	Maria Luisa	1901,09,15 (1921) 1923	Chincolco (out of valley)	--	--	--
8	Maria Jesus	1915,23,26,29, 32,34,37	Chincolco	--	--	--
9	Maria del Socorro	1927,30,37	Chincolco	1907	+	--
10	Maria	1934,36	Chincolco	1911	+	+
11	Maria Primitiva	1939	Chincolco	1911	--	--
12	Maria Claudina	1953	Chincolco	1929	--	--
13	Maria Ines	1956	Chincolco	1940	+	--
14	Maria Eduvina	1958 (twins)	Chincolco	1941	+	--

Source: Family pedigrees.

*Mother's second maiden name (in Spanish, apellido materno).

Christian and family names were lumped together. Next, the clumps were examined for obvious impossibilities (e.g. births strung over thirty or more years). In the example, there were four groups of Maria's at this stage: 2-3; 4-5; 6; and 10. The remaining mothers with second Christian names clustered as in the Table. Then a segregating process was applied to split down these clusters on the basis of available discordant information (mother's birthdate, second family name, conflicting witnesses, etc.). For children born prior to 1900, birthplace information was the principal criteria. An arbitrary rule was applied to nineteenth-century children: unless there was a match on two Christian names, offspring born in different parts of the valley were assigned to different mothers. This caused clusters 2-3 and 4-5 to split. Where ages of mothers were given, the maximum absolute difference permitted was two years. In the example, no disaggregations occurred on this variable. Nor were there any splits caused by the second family name. After completing the breaking-down cycle, renewed links were attempted with positive auxiliary information. Joining family 6 to 7 would have weakened the already existing links (on name and age), but 10 and 11 continued as possible links. If the mother of one of the children in 10 had been referred to as "Primitiva" or had the second family name been present or the grandmother appeared as the witness for the inscription of the child in family 11, the two families could have been confidently combined into one. The final arrangement is contentious. After this stage was completed, mothers with second Christian names were compared with mothers with the same given names to see if there might be sufficient positive information for further linkages. In the example no new links were made. This illustration indicates that most of the clusters have been made with rather strong links. Nevertheless, uncertainty remains about the final disposition of 10-11. These ambiguities must have ramifications for interpreting patterns of illegitimacy.

The repercussions of this uncertainty become even greater when linking illegitimate children to a mother who later marries. Birth rank is a particularly important control in analyzing both infant mortality and birth intervals--but the analysis is complicated by the proportion of uncertain linkages. For children who were legitimized at marriage, these difficulties are successfully resolved, but a substantial portion of children were attributed to mothers who later married without legitimizing all of their children (Table A1.3). Although the linking algorithm should err toward excess exclusion, some children were probably incorrectly attributed. Consequently, the distinction between brides with premarital births and those without is speculative to some degree.

TABLE A1.3
Children's birthdate compared with parents' marriage date

Period of Birth	Children Born After Parent's Marriage (1)	Children Legitimated at Parents' Marriage (2)	Children Attributed to Parent Later Marrying (3)	2/(2+3) Percent
1840-1864	5377	0	985	0.0
1865-1884	3155	1	699	0.1
1885-1914	4006	228	849	21.2
1915-1929	1247	323	320	50.2
1930-1939	1176	220	212	50.9
1940-1949	1310	178	189	48.5
1950-1959	1384	169	206	45.1
1960-1964	695	69	55	55.6
1965-1970	208	51	29	63.8

Dataset: Births.

NOTE: After 1915, the Bureau encouraged parents to legitimize children born before marriage.

TERMINATING FAMILY HISTORIES WITH THE 1970 CENSUS

A third bias peculiar to this study is the way in which family histories are terminated for those still lacking, by April 1970, the death of the first spouse to expire. Two strategies are customarily available for tying off reconstitution studies: (1) continue to search for events of reconstituted families for some sixty years beyond the conclusion date, or (2) cap off unfinished families by tying them into a manuscript census. The principal difficulty lies in determining which families still reside in the community at the termination date. That bit of information saves the last cohort for analytical purposes. If the study simply ends abruptly, an entire generation of families must be discarded; otherwise, those in the last fifty year cohort would be biased toward premature terminations. Neither option, however, was available in this study. Chilean law prohibits the use of official nominative census information by people not associated with the National Statistical Institute. My proposal, to subcontract census personnel to link the enumerated population into the reconstituted families and then excise the names, was rejected by the Institute. The risk of violating the confidentiality of the census was considered too great. Nevertheless, the Institute graciously made available coded transcripts of the enumerators' sheets with the names deleted.

Once the family histories were completely reconstituted,

it took some time to develop a statistical linking algorithm which would yield satisfying results. The goal was to save the maximum number of histories without linking families which had actually left the community. Rates calculated from poorly linked families would be downwardly biased because the denominator of the rate would be inflated without the possibility of any increase in the numerator. For example, in calculating fertility rates, the numbers of mothers at risk would be augmented by the statistical linkages, but births to linked mothers actually residing outside the community could not appear in the life histories and consequently the estimates would be correspondingly lowered.

After considerable analysis of the histories and enumerators' sheets, the following algorithm was developed. Only legally married families could be considered. Since migrating spouses cause the whole problem, those with a record of moving about were also excluded. To reduce the arbitrariness of the links three bits of information--the ages of both spouses in 1970 and information on total births--were used to create small pools from which linked families were drawn by lot. Table A1.4 indicates the application of this algorithm to the information available in the two data sets. Step six of the algorithm is elaborated in Tables A1.5 and A1.6. The ratios in the first Table indicate the proportions within each pair of age cohorts declared to be linked. Note that for younger ages, selection by birth information tended to exclude links; older spouses were not as affected by this factor, because with only a very small fraction of families still in the area it was highly probable that at least one family with the appropriate number of children could be found in the longitudinal data set. For example, there were six family histories with wives aged 20-24 and husbands aged 30-34 in 1970, but only two of these could be linked (Table A1.5, row 2, column 3), notwithstanding five enumerated pairs of spouses with these ages (Table A1.6, same cell). Four families were not linked because they failed to agree with the three census families on brood size. At the opposite extreme, there were eleven histories with spouses aged 70-74 in 1970, but there was only one family with these same characteristics in the census. For all groups with spouses less than fifty-five years old, the fraction of histories linked hovers above 50 percent. The rather low linkage ratios for young, enumerated spouses can be explained by two considerations: illegitimacy and migration. Given that one in five registered births in the community in the late sixties were illegitimate, the percentage of consensual unions (1 percent) in the census seems much too low. Perhaps many of these couples considered themselves married but had not yet legally registered the fact. Similarly, migration data is notoriously unreliable. Possibly some of these young couples married outside the community, migrated in, and appeared in the census as stable residents,

TABLE A1.4
Algorithm for linking family histories to 1970 census enumerators' sheets

Family Histories		Enumerated Spouses	
Criteria	Number	Criteria	Number
Total family histories	2662	Total enumerated families	853
1. Exclude parents not married in study area	-873	1. Exclude unmarried spouses	-10
2. Exclude families with fathers born outside or residing outside community at marriage	-872	2. Exclude fathers born out or residing out in 1965 or absent from family at census	-192
3. Exclude families with mothers residing out at marriage	-43	3. Exclude families with mothers residing out in 1965 or absent at census	-89
4. Exclude parents lacking birthdate information	-46	4. Exclude parents lacking birthdate information	0
5. Exclude families with one parent dead prior to 1970 census	-175	5. Exclude widowed spouses	-137
Total family histories with exclusions	653	Total enumerated families with exclusions	425
6. Group families by five-year birth cohorts on the basis of both parents' ages in 1970		6. Group families by five-year birth cohorts on the basis of both parents' ages in 1970	
7. Within each age group form clusters by number of children born prior to census date		7. Within each age group form clusters by declared children ever born (group 7-8; 9 or more)	
8. Calculate the probability ratio for each cluster (number of census families/number of family histories). Select or reject as determined by a table of random numbers. Selected histories are assigned a code, indicating in observation at census date.		8. Calculate the probability ratio for each cluster (number of census families/number of family histories). Select or reject as determined by a table of random numbers. Selected histories are assigned a code, indicating in observation at census date.	

TABLE A1.5
Ratio of linked families to life histories by ages of spouses

Age of Wife	Age of Husband 20–24	25–29	30–34	34–39	40–44	45–49	50–54	55–59	60–64	65–69	70–74	75+	Totals	% Linked
15–19	4/4	3/4											7/8	87
20–24	6/9	11/17	2/6	2/5			1/1						22/38	58
25–29	1/3	14/17	18/28	10/13	2/6	2/2					1/1		48/70	69
30–34		5/6	12/22	20/33	7/13	3/5	0/1		1/1				48/81	59
35–39	0/1	1/1	2/5	15/22	16/20	6/13	6/7	0/1					46/70	66
40–44				3/6	8/15	16/19	6/10	3/7	1/2	1/2		1/1	39/62	63
45–49			0/2	2/5	1/6	7/16	13/23	6/10	3/7				32/69	46
50–54				0/2	1/2	4/6	7/9	4/11	3/8	2/4	0/1		21/43	49
55–59						0/1	2/7	2/18	11/14	6/8	1/5		22/53	42
60–64						0/1	0/1	5/12	5/15	9/19	1/3	0/2	20/53	38
65–69								0/3	1/4	4/20	2/14	1/7	8/48	17
70–74							0/1	0/1		0/3	1/11	0/17	1/33	3
75+								0/1			0/1	1/23	1/25	4
Totals	11/17	34/45	34/63	52/86	35/62	38/63	35/60	20/64	25/51	22/56	6/36	3/50	315/653	
% Linked	65	76	54	60	56	60	58	31	49	39	17	6		48

TABLE A1.6
Ratio of linked families to census families by ages of spouses

	Age of Husband												
Age of Wife	20-24	25-29	30-34	34-39	40-44	45-49	50-54	55-59	60-64	65-69	70-74	75+	Totals	% Linked
15-19	4/9	3/4											7/13	54
20-24	6/13	11/25	2/5	2/2			1/1						22/46	48
25-29	1/1	14/34	18/27	10/12	2/2	2/2					1/1		48/79	61
30-34	0/2	5/5	12/14	20/21	7/10	3/3	0/1	0/1	1/1				48/58	83
35-39		1/1	2/2	15/26	16/19	6/8	6/6						46/62	74
40-44				3/3	8/10	16/17	6/6	3/3	1/2	1/1		1/1	39/43	91
45-49				2/2	1/2	7/10	13/13	6/7	3/3				32/37	86
50-54				0/1	1/2	4/4	7/7	4/4	3/4	2/2	0/1		21/25	82
55-59							2/2	2/2	11/11	6/6	1/1	0/1	22/23	96
60-64						0/1		5/5	5/5	9/9	1/1	0/1	20/22	91
65-69					0/1			0/1	1/1	4/4	2/2	1/1	8/10	80
70-74										0/1	1/1		1/2	50
75+								0/1		0/1		1/3	1/5	20
Totals	11/25	34/69	34/48	52/67	35/46	38/45	35/36	20/24	25/27	22/24	6/7	3/7	315/425	
% Linked	44	49	71	78	76	84	97	83	93	92	86	43		74

whether or not their residency histories were reported accurately.

In conclusion, the technical sewing up of family histories in reconstitution studies is absolutely necessary to be able to analyze the demographic experiences of the last generation. The threads used for finishing up that group in this study are of very poor quality indeed. Random links are weak substitutes for nominal ones. But given the importance of analyzing the more recent trends, a probabilistic finish is better than simply leaving the edges frayed. Notwithstanding a less than 50 percent chance of forming a true link for most groups, the algorithm should contribute to choosing the demographically appropriate family within each cluster.

UNDERREGISTRATION OF BIRTHS

Finally, a third, and perhaps the most intractable problem which tends to erupt incessantly in reconstitution studies is the rate of omissions from the vital registers. The coverage of the national registration system has long been a depressing subject amongst Chilean scholars. The Statistical Annuals of the late nineteenth century graphically portray the sharp, prolonged dip in registered events which began in 1885 with the change from a religious to a civil registration system. For many years the annual demographic publications included cursory remarks that some undetermined proportion of events were not being registered.

To compensate for underrecording births during the first eighty years of its existence the Statistical Bureau simply reported births by year of registration instead of by year of occurrence. In 1928 this practice was modified. Infants registered at less than two years of age were tabulated as being born in the year of registration. Finally, in 1952 the Bureau began the curious practice of reporting by year of occurrence only those births registered within three months of the calendar year of parturition. At the same time the Bureau set the estimated rate of underregistration of live births at 5 percent.[3]

These arbitrary official adjustments indicate little about the magnitude of omissions. Hugo Behm has applied a more intuitively appealing method to the birth data for the period 1930-1960. He simply retabulated all births by year of occurrence regardless of registration date. While noting that this procedure yielded only minimum omissions since obviously varying numbers of births were never recorded at all, he emphasized that the retabulations typically exceeded the official estimates by several percent. In 1963, a senior researcher at the United Nations Demographic Center in Santiago used a statistical method, a cohort population balance sheet, to produce a third series of estimates. These assessments lead to similar conclusions. The percentage of unreported births has been

TABLE A1.7
Three estimates of unrecorded births: Chile, 1930-1960 (in percentages)

Period	Official[a]	Assignment to Year of Birth[b]	Population Balance Sheet[c]
1930-1939	13.8	13.4	19.2
1940-1951	10.3	12.7	14.3
1952-1954	5.0	11.7	10.8
1954-1960	4.0	8.8	8.1

[a]Calculated from data in Instituto Nacional de Estadística, Demografía, Ano 1966, p. 62 and Behm, Mortalidad infantíl, p. 35.

[b]Hugo Behm, Mortalidad infantíl y nivél de vida (Santiago, 1962), p. 35.

[c]Johannes L. Sadie, "Población y mano de obra de Chile, 1930-1975," in Chile (Santiago, 1969), pp. 18-19.

extremely high in the past and was still substantial as late as 1960 (Table A1.7).

The implications of such high levels of omissions for a family reconstitution study are unsettling. Nevertheless, it should be apparent that these estimates are based on untested hypotheses and not empirical analysis. Behm's procedure in particular inadvertently includes an unknown, but perhaps substantial, proportion of late, repeated registrations. Until the late fifties duplicated registrations for legitimizing or recognizing natural children (very frequent given the high rates of illegitimacy), name changes, correction of errors, etc., were apparently repeated in the birth series. Moreover, all of these estimates apply to the Chilean population as an aggregate. They are gross estimates, a summation of the errors for all regions and social classes.

Certainly at the national level, this substantial rate of omission should discourage high expectations from the Chilean registers. One should realize that much of the underreporting reflects not so much the education and civic pride of the Chilean people as the legal importance of each child to its parents and the inconvenience of registering an event. The lives of legitimate children of modest laborers living in a small valley with a mild climate and a conveniently located registration office might be very well recorded; however, information about illegitimate children born to self-supporting mothers with registration necessitating considerable effort to pay bus fare, overcome the vagaries of the weather, meet the economic needs of the family, and cope with the whims of registration

TABLE A1.8
Underregistration of live births: selected provinces, 1950, 1957

	Omission Rate (percentages)		
Province	1950	1957	Registered Live Births in 1957
Antofagasta	3.5	7.2	3,797
Aconcagua	5.1	4.5	4,759
Santiago	9.7	8.5	78,770
Colchagua	13.7	7.9	5,780
Linares	21.4	13.4	5,731
Cautín	24.8	25.4	10,401
Magallanes	3.4	3.6	1,782
Chile	11.9	5.6	273,153

Source: Behm, *Mortalidad infantíl*, pp. 35, 40.

NOTE: Petorca Valley is located in Aconcagua province.

officers might be much less complete. Behm's data on estimated underreporting by provinces indicate widely varying rates (Table A1.8). If within specific regions much of the underregistration should prove to be restricted to defined subsets of the population, the reliability of small group statistics could be salvaged by separating the poorly registered.

The empirical analysis of registration practices is hampered because all assessments must be limited to discovering registration inconsistencies rather than determining the actual proportion of unregistered events. Two tests are applied to the Petorca birth records: discovery of the number of Petorcans inscribed in the death registers whose births were not recorded, and analysis of the relative tardiness of birth registrations on the supposition that inscription lag is closely correlated with omissions. Table A1.9 indicates that since 1885, as one might expect, there has been a substantial drop in the percentage of unrecorded births. The surprising discovery in this Table is that as early as 1895-1909 the level of underreporting for children born to parents previously married in the study area reached an astonishingly low level (0.8-2.3 percent). During the same period natural children and infants born to parents who married outside the community had much higher rates of omission (4.5-13.6 percent). These estimates are only observed minima. There must have been many other children who had neither their deaths nor births recorded.[4]

A better indication of the proportion of unregistered

TABLE A1.9
Birth underregistration estimated from burials: Petorca, 1885-1969

Birth Cohort	Number of Deaths Without Birth Inscriptions		Percent of Total Births		Percent of Total Deaths	
	Born After	Other	Born After	Other	Born After	Other
1885-1894	50	121	3.8	8.2	10.8	27.3
1895-1909	15	87	0.8	4.5	2.3	13.6
1910-1929	8	54	0.4	2.6	1.4	7.7
1930-1949	12	19	0.4	1.0	2.0	4.7
1950-1969	12	29	0.4	2.0	3.2	12.6

Dataset: Births, Deaths.

NOTE: "Born After"--child born after parents' marriage in study area.

births can be obtained by examining the distribution of omissions by age at death (Table A1.10). During the decade 1885-1894, 50.6 percent of the infants dying within the first year of life and born to parents not married in the community had no corresponding birth slip. The proportion declines to 21 percent for those dying at age one and 14 percent for deaths beyond the second birthday. Over the decades a substantial decline in the proportion of deaths lacking birth slips occurred. The pattern is similar for infants born after the parents' marriage in the valley; however, the omission rate is roughly one-half of the other group. The three indicators for each group all yield diverse percentages of unrecorded births because of differing sensitivities to the lag in recording births. In fact, the percentage of unrecorded births calculated from infant deaths essentially reflects the birth registration lag. Of the eighty-one deaths from 1885-1894 lacking a birth slip (for other families), fifty-five occurred within one month of birth. During this same period only 30 percent of births were recorded within the first month following parturition. Underrecordings at later ages of death are much less disturbed by the delay in inscribing births. While the third indicator, percentage not registered of those dying at age two and above, is virtually unaffected by the birth registration lag, the observed percentages are probably understated because of heavier out-migration at young adult ages. The best indicator for estimating the proportion of completely unrecoverable births (i.e. with no recorded birth or death) and the one least affected by migration and late inscriptions, would seem to be that based on deaths at age one year and above. It is that ratio which is used for adjusting age specific fertility rates (see Table 5.6).

The information in Table A1.10 represents a considerable advance in understanding the pattern of omissions from Chilean birth registers. Without consideration of the parents' status, 40 percent of the infant deaths in the period 1885-1894 were not preceded by a birth inscription. (If this pattern was general, national infant mortality rates may be considerably overstated for the late nineteenth and early twentieth centuries.) While this percentage dropped drastically in succeeding periods, it has recently risen to almost 7 percent of deaths within the first year of life.

These figures represent the proportion of detectable omissions. How can the underrecording of births of those who did not die be assessed? If the likelihood of registering a child's death is independent of the recording of its birth, then the percentage of observed underreporting could be applied directly to the observed births as a correction factor. Since it is very likely that parents indisposed to register births would also tend to neglect the registration of infant deaths, this adjustment should be considered a minimum.

TABLE A1.10
Deaths with missing birth inscriptions by age at death and family type: Petorca, 1885-1969

Age at Death	1885-1894	1895-1909	1910-1934	1935-1949	1950-1969
			Number of Cases		
Born after parents' marriage in study area					
1-11 months	35	10	4	4	6
1 year	5	1	3	4	1
2+ years	10	4	2	3	0
Other families					
1-11 months	81	46	27	6	29
1 year	13	9	10	5	0
2+ years	27	32	22	3	0
All Families					
1-11 months	116	56	31	10	35
1 year	18	10	13	9	1
2+ years	37	36	24	6	0
			As Percentage of All Deaths		
Born after parents' marriage in study area					
1-11 months	24.6	4.0	1.1	1.3	1.9
1 year	9.1	1.2	3.9	5.8	2.6
2+ years	3.8	1.4	0.8	3.2	--
Other families					
1-11 months	50.6	15.6	5.5	2.8	14.1
1 year	20.7	9.6	11.1	11.9	--
2+ years	14.3	12.6	9.1	7.7	--
All families					
1-11 months	38.4	10.3	3.6	1.9	6.7
1 year	15.3	5.6	7.8	8.1	2.0
2+ years	8.2	6.7	4.9	4.5	--

Dataset: Births, Deaths.

These data also demonstrate that most of the omissions are confined to children born to families who did not marry in the community. Even in the earliest periods the magnitude of omissions is manageable for substantive analysis. In succeeding years the proportion of omissions for the prime reconstitutable families is very small. In fact, the absolute number is so tiny that it could easily be within the domain of reconstitution errors.

Additional support for this auspicious conclusion can be obtained from an analysis of the lag between parturition and the recording of the birth event (Figure A1.1). The birth inscription pattern for infants born to parents after their marriage in Petorca indicates that as early as 1900-1904, over 90 percent of all births in the community were inscribed within two months of birth. This inscription record compares poorly with rural eighteenth-century French parishes, where almost all infants were baptized within only three days of birth. On the other hand, civil registration in Petorca is somewhat better than that reported for the English parish studied by Wrigley.[5] However, throughout much of the nineteenth century baptisms in Petorca occurred tardily indeed. During the period of ecclesiastical registration at least 20 percent of births to parents who married in the parish either were never baptized or were inscribed after a lapse of two or more years. Consequently, demographic estimates for the nineteenth century must be considered approximate in the extreme. On the other hand, the civil system achieved a high level of efficiency within a decade or so of its founding.

For children born to unmarried parents or to those who married elsewhere, birth registration was much delayed (Figure A1.1). Greater proportions either were never inscribed or were registered at older ages. Beginning in the 1930s birth registration deteriorated slightly as parents delayed inscriptions in the first month. However, there was little effect on the proportion of inscriptions occurring within two months of birth.

The changing degree of birth omissions and the relative tardiness of inscriptions over the past century has some unfortunate implications for the analysis of fertility. Clearly, given the degree of underregistration some adjustment to the observed rates is necessary; consequently, analysis must be restricted to measures which are correctable with the underregistration ratios. These considerations restrict analysis to age-specific marital fertility rates. The means of correction for these measures are straightforward: simply inflate the observed rate by the estimated omission ratio. Other sophisticated and very interesting fertility indicators--the distribution of birth intervals by parity, age of mother at the birth of various parities, etc.--must be ignored because there are no satisfying means for correcting the observed figures throughout the period studied (1840-1969). (The omission pattern is sufficiently small in the twentieth century

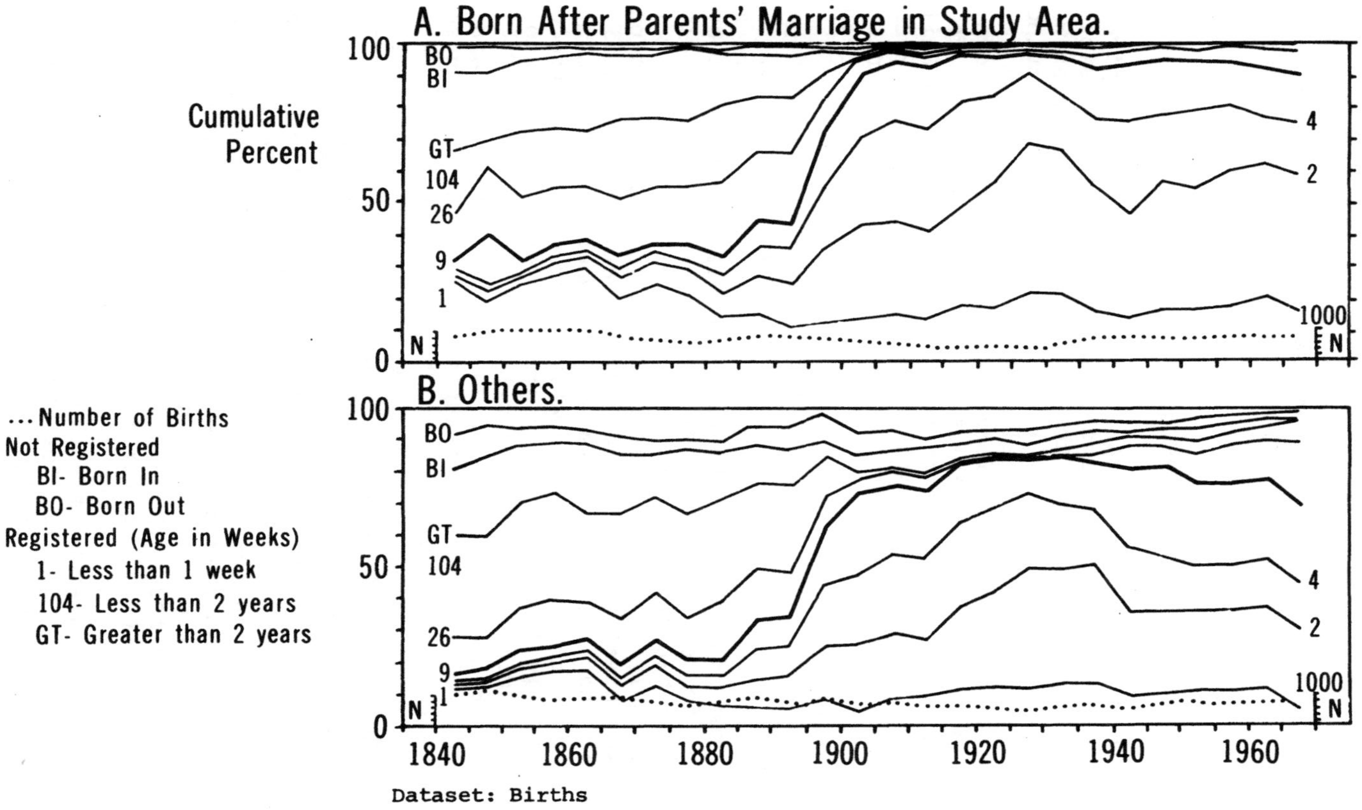

Figure A1.1 Birth registration lag by birth cohorts and family type

that these measures could be used with some confidence.) A key natality indicator, age-specific legitimate fertility rates, are readily adjustable over the entire span of the study and for this reason have been used throughout the discussion on fertility change and natality differentials.

THE QUALITY OF MARRIAGE RECORDS

Researchers of Chilean population dynamics typically shun discussion of marriage trends as either impossible or irrelevant. A glance at the sharp drop in marriages with the initiation of the civil registration system convinces most researchers that legal marriage is only a hazy reflection of real family formation patterns. Therefore, with no information other than inscribed marriages, few attempt to assess these matters in any detail--the Chilean marriage data being considered virtually useless for demographic purposes.[6] Given the very substantial attention to marriage patterns here, the quality of marriage records must be examined.

Prior to 1850 marriage inscriptions for Petorca parish suffer from lax procedures and poor preservation. For the period 1830-1849, over 1400 couples appear in the marriage records, but both banns documents and marriage acts survive for only one-half of these. A marriage act alone was locatable for about 40 percent; for the remaining 10 percent only the banns documents remain. The situation improves greatly after 1850. From that year only a tiny fraction have incomplete sets of documents, and in almost every case the omission probably occurred because the couple actually failed to marry (refusal of the church to waive impediments, death, etc.).

In 1885 with the establishment of civil registers, marriage records became disrupted again; however, these shortcomings were overcome in the reconstitution work by continuing to use marriages from the parish books for another decade (through 1896). In fact, the Petorca records themselves suffered very little from the change; most of the decline occurred for people living in Hierro Viejo. This situation contrasts sharply with the national trends where there developed considerable disparity between custom and law, confirming the worries of the ecclesiastical authorities who feared a breakdown of morals with the establishment of civil registration. In Petorca the age at marriage rose for both sexes, as did the proportion of brides with natural children. Later, a decline in absolute numbers of marriages (for the 1900-1914 cohort) is a result of the dismemberment of Hierro Viejo district (reincorporated in 1930). For the same cohort, the lower proportion of young brides and the greater percentage of brides with natural children confirms that marriage customs and law diverged more than ever.

In addition to these general tendencies, the movement of marriages from year to year demands a closer analysis to ascertain registration efficiency. Violent fluctuations in the marriage series must be examined to determine the correspondence between registered marriages and the social realities of family formation. To what extent are excess marriages in peak years a catching-up of delayed inscriptions, the sporadic inclusion of families customarily estranged from the system, or simply fluctuations responding to short-term demographic and economic conditions? If it is impossible to determine the precise relative importance of these factors, certain inferences may be drawn on the basis of the bride's age, previous marital status, and premarital pregnancy history. An increase in the proportion of younger brides in peak years suggests economic and social circumstances facilitating earlier marriage, but not a faulty registration system. A greater proportion of elderly brides with more children born prior to wedlock indicate postponed registration, or the sporadic enticement into the registration net of families initiated several years earlier. In order to establish a norm against which peaks may be compared, the average number and type of marriages in the immediately preceding three-year period is used.

As early as 1857 peak marriage years probably reflected real changes in the frequency of marriage rather than changing administrative efficiency. For each of the four marriage peaks after 1850--1857, 1889, 1896, and 1933--there is a general dampening of fluctuations and indications of consistent coverage (Table A1.11). Sophisticated analysis is not required to demonstrate that marriage peaks before the 1850s were induced by administrative considerations rather than social or economic ones. Two-thirds of the marriages registered during 1838 took place during the pastoral visit of the Archbishop-Elect.[7] During the peak of 1848 fully one-half of all marriages were celebrated in a single month. More marriages were registered in that year than in the immediately preceding triennium. Brides in 1848 were also relatively older and more likely to have had children before marriage. The low percentage of remarriages implies that a mortality or subsistence crisis was not a causal factor. Clearly many of the 1848 brides received the marital blessings of the Church only after cohabitating with their mates for some years and as a result of extraordinary efforts by the parish priest to carry a missionary effort directly to the people.

The pattern for later peak years differs markedly from that of 1848. The peaks are much lower, the monthly concentration virtually disappears, and the demographic characteristics of the brides more closely approximate the pattern for the respective triennium. The 1857 peak seems to have resulted not from the sudden registration of families initiated several years before, but from an abrupt

TABLE A1.11
Bumper and average marriage years

	1845-1847	1848	1854-1856	1857	1886-1888	1889	1893-1895	1896	1930-1932	1933
Marriages per year	43.3	149	49.0	85	47.3	106	42.0	94	48.3	76
Ratio	3.4		1.7		2.2		2.2		1.6	
Bride's Age at Marriage (percent)										
-19	22	23	19	25	16	18	18	12	30	24
20-24	32	30	41	34	31	20	25	22	34	27
25-29	36	34	27	34	26	36	33	40	16	21
30-	10	14	13	6	27	26	24	26	20	28
Bride's Premarital Pregnancy Experience (percent)										
Prenuptial Conception	16	11	13	20	14	15	14	12	10	6
Prenuptial Birth	42	53	41	23	41	40	34	57	31	52
No Prenuptial Conception	43	36	46	57	46	46	53	30	59	43
Bride's Marital Order (percent)										
First	90	96	97	99	94	91	94	88	95	93
Other	10	4	3	1	6	9	6	12	5	7

Dataset: Marriages.

NOTE: Percentages exclude women of unknown age and marital status. Data on age and pregnancy refers to first marriages only. Triennial figures are averages.

increase in the frequency of marriage in that year. When compared with brides of the 1854-1856 period, 1857 brides were younger, less likely to have born children out of wedlock, and more likely to have been pregnant at marriage. In fact, there was an absolute decrease in marriages by older women aged thirty or more years, and by women who had born illegitimate children. The relative distributions suggest that by roughly the middle of the nineteenth century marriage sacraments had acquired the character of a popularly accepted system which approximated the family formation customs of the valley. Certainly campaigns to take marriage sacraments to parishioners, like those of 1838 and 1848, were no longer necessary.

The marriage surge of 1889 seems to have been a response to the 1888 cholera epidemic, and the generally hard times of 1887-1888. Rather than a systematic failure to register marriages over a long period of time, remarriage by widows and the higher percentage of women marrying a few years later than customary (ages 25-29) indicate a response to improving social, economic, and demographic conditions.

Characteristics of marriages for the year 1896 are more contradictory. The age and marital status data of brides present a pattern of variations which could arise from a short delay in marriage as a response to momentarily adverse economic and demographic conditions (slightly older ages at marriage and a higher proportion with premarital births). However, there are quantitative indications of some registration problems as well. The higher percentage of women bearing children before marriage and the much larger average number of natural children (mean of 2.9 children born before marriage of brides aged 25+ years in 1896 versus only 2.2 for the triennium) imply that in that year women were making a legal step to formalize a family situation started several years earlier.

Finally, in 1933, there is once again a larger proportion of older brides and a greater proportion with natural children. This technically unsettling finding is offset to some extent by the comparatively low value of the ratio and the fact that much of the increase came from in-migrants rather than from Petorcans per se. The average number of marriages by native Petorcans increased only 30 percent while those by outsiders more than doubled.

In general, this comparison of bumper marriage years and normal periods supports the thesis that officially registered marriages reflected family formation customs in a systematic way. The point is to demonstrate a rather slow evolution of administrative efficiency rather than to argue that people only bore children within marriage. Marriage, then, has not been a sporadic phenomenon dependent upon the zeal of administrators or abrupt bureaucratic inducements. On the contrary, the decision to obtain a legal marriage seems to have been related systematically to informal family formation customs.

THE REGISTRATION OF DEATHS

In contrast to the numerous critiques of national birth statistics, assessment of Chilean death registration has been virtually unknown until recently. Lacking empirical indications, specialists have been compelled to suggest possible minor underrecording, decreasing with improvements in education and transportation. In 1973 these crude intuitions were shattered with the publication of the results of an exhaustive investigation of infant mortality sponsored by the Pan American Health Organization.[8] The researchers sampled the death records of Santiago hospitals and then searched the vital events books in an attempt to empirically assess the rate of omission for deaths occurring in hospitals. Their conclusions are astonishing. As many as 80 percent of infant deaths occurring within one hour of birth were not officially registered. Overall, some 56 percent of infant deaths in the sample had not been reported to the registrars.

Before one despairs about using the Chilean death data, it should be emphasized that this extraordinary rate of omissions may reflect conditions peculiar to large Chilean cities: that is, extremely crowded hospitals with procedures for burying unclaimed bodies at the hospitals' expense, exorbitant private burial fees even for newborn infants, long lines and short hours at the civil registry offices, and the failure of hospital staff to file prepared death reports. A national survey designed to empirically evaluate the degree of omission in the death registers is necessary to reduce the confused speculation over the reliability of the officially collected death information.

Working with mortality data for the Petorca Valley is the most difficult of all. Underregistration of infant deaths was so high in the nineteenth century that the rate is impossible to quantify precisely. The problem for the parish era is further complicated by an inability to link deaths of children to family histories. Even underregistration of adult deaths is known to have occurred. People wishing to remarry sometimes had to resort to the use of witnesses who vouched for one's widowhood. Priests readily accepted these testimonies because of the notorious shortcomings of the burial registers. (One man boldly used this technique while his first wife was still alive and resident in the parish!)

Twentieth-century data is more reliable, but the short period prevents one from saying much about adult mortality since most of the subjects were still alive when the study concluded. Death data for infants and children are much more reliable and manageable regardless of the method opted for. In general, the quality of the death registers for this century is sufficiently high that one may confidently conclude that the mortality trends presented above are very close to the actual ones.

The following critique focuses on three stages of the life cycle--adulthood, infancy, and childhood--because procedures for detecting omissions have features particular to each. No mortality estimates for adults have been presented here because the basic data is too skimpy. The family history method limits itself to considering adults who marry in the study area (i.e. marriage date determines entry into observation, exit date is date of death or an attributed date in cases where the precise death date is unknown). Adult mortality for Petorca is virtually unanalyzable because actual death dates are known for only a small fraction of the total married population (Table A1.12). For studies of European communities the small proportion of unknown deaths are simply distributed according to various suppositions to generate extreme bounds. However, in this case the proportion of unknowns is so great that the exercise becomes futile; the range is so great that the estimates contribute nothing.[9]

However, infant mortality data is much less frustrating to work with. During the parish era the underrecording of infant deaths was so extreme that often infant mortality rates were almost as low as those for children aged one year. After the institution of a civil system the ratio rose as high as five to one (that is, the infant mortality rate became five times the rate for one year olds). Perhaps as many as two-thirds of the infant deaths were omitted from the parish burial registers.

With civil registration, death inscriptions improved substantially in terms of both registration completeness and detail of entries. Two principal techniques have been developed for analyzing omissions of infant burials through analysis of family histories. One strategy, favored by English historians, proposes a model distribution of deaths at various ages during the first year of life; the other, elaborated by French historical demographers, analyzes birth intervals according to the survival status of the first of two infants forming the interval.[10]

It should be apparent from the analysis of birth registration that the omission rate depends upon the particular subset of families being analyzed. The more sophisticated techniques proposed by the French must be limited to infants born to couples who married in the study area, while the English approach may be used for the entire population. The critique which follows focuses exclusively on the prime histories because these form the basis for the substantive analysis in earlier chapters.

Wrigley suggests that if fewer than 50 percent of inscribed infant deaths are listed at less than one month of age it is likely due to failure to register a corresponding proportion of neonatal deaths. Except for recent years, the Petorca data fall within the plausible range (Table A1.13). Nevertheless, the method is not particularly

TABLE A1.12
Marriages and known death dates

Petorca Males Birth Cohort	Total Marriages	Percent with Death Dates
1820-1839	1020	36.1
1840-1859	881	33.5
1860-1879	805	28.6
1880-1894	410	34.4
1895-1909	532	21.2
1910-1924	470	9.6
1925-1939	459	2.2
1940-1954	162	0.6
Colyton (both sexes)	345	65.8
Crulai (males)	261	79.7

Sources: Marriages Dataset; Wrigley, "Mortality in Pre-industrial England," p. 554; Gautier and Henry, La population de Crulai, p. 179.

convincing for several reasons. First, it is insensitive to omissions which are independent of age. Secondly, stillbirths are often impossible to distinguish from infant deaths. This fact tends to boost the proportion of deaths during the first month of life. Finally, recent research has demonstrated that there is much variability in death rates within the first year of life. The actual pattern is particularly dependent upon breast feeding and weaning customs and the incidence and severity of certain illnesses peculiar to infancy. Knodel and Hinter argue that the pattern is distinctly different for breast fed and nonbreast fed infants, with the former having a greater concentration of deaths shortly after birth and, for the latter, a surge of deaths occur around the age at which premature weaning takes place.[11] In a study of a Malaysian population, Smith found the proportion of late infant and early childhood mortality to be much higher than for most European and contemporary populations.[12] Perhaps within specific European cultural areas with long lactation periods there was a fairly rigid mortality pattern during the first year of life; however, this proposal hardly seems sufficient for rejecting or accepting figures from a distinctly different region.

A second ratio relationship proposed by Hollingsworth seems even less useful. He argues that deaths in the first three months should be about five times as great as those in the last nine. His reasoning was apparently based on a single, very particular example: Crulai parish

TABLE A1.13
Distribution of mortality within first year of life (ages in months)

	Infant Mortality Rate	Deaths 0-2 (a)	Deaths 3-11 (b)	Ratio a/b	Deaths 0 (c)	Deaths 0-11 (d)	c/d (%)
Tourouvre							
1680-1689	288	108	30	3.60	67	138	48.6
1700-1710	298	114	36	3.17	82	150	54.7
1720-1729	266	105	24	4.38	80	129	62.0
1740-1749	273	85	17	5.00	71	102	69.6
1760-1769	174	56	20	2.80	46	76	60.5
Crulai							
1688-1719	236	158	38	4.16	128	196	65.3
1720-	172	118	17	6.94	105	135	77.8
Colyton							
1438-1499	108	165	63	2.54	119	228	52.2
1600-1649	81	160	81	1.98	100	241	41.5
1650-1699	79	105	53	1.98	73	158	46.2
1700-1749	98	83	48	1.73	57	131	43.5
1750-1837	72	168	101	1.66	117	269	43.5
Cocos-Keeling							
1888-1912	377	--	--	--	120	316	38.0
1913-1917	188	--	--	--	17	34	50.0
1918-1942	90	--	--	--	58	147	39.5
Petorca							
1885-1914	137	540	220	2.39	404	785	51.5
1915-1929	175	305	112	2.72	237	417	56.8
1930-1939	142	202	86	2.34	155	288	53.8
1940-1949	123	163	87	1.87	124	250	49.6
1950-1959	119	160	105	1.52	120	265	45.3
1960-1969	93	110	69	1.59	74	179	41.3

Sources: At Risk Dataset; Wrigley, "Mortality in Pre-industrial England," p. 565; Gautier and Henry, La population de Crulai, p. 268; Charbonneau, Tourouvre-au-Perche, pp. 389-408; Hollingsworth, "The Importance of the Quality," pp. 423-425; Smith, "The Cocos-Keeling Islands," pp. 120-122.

NOTE: Cocos-Keeling data specifically excludes stillbirths; Colyton data include children with "manufactured" birthdates.

where over 75 percent of infant deaths occurred within one month of birth. Other French studies have not produced a ratio as high as that for Crulai (Table A1.13). Applying the proportions to the Petorca data would yield infant mortality rates of 237, 282, 254, 257, 283, and 215 for the six periods from 1885 through 1969 (with death omissions varying from 75 to 130 percent). This pattern is not credible and must be rejected. The ratio suffers from the same shortcomings as Wrigley's. The one seems to find underregistration everywhere while the other is not very powerful.

The Henry method is theoretically much more elegant. It is based on a relatively simple, yet highly plausible proposition: in a natural fertility regime, conception occurs much sooner following an infant death than when the preceding infant survives. Therefore, a comparison of intervals in which the preceding infant is a known survivor with those in which survivorship is unknown indicates the relative degree of omission in the death registers. There is a presumption that death and birth omissions are unrelated (otherwise intervals for the unknown category would be lengthened by omission of births). Finally, efficiency of the method increases as the proportion of those with unknown survival status declines.

Almost none of these relationships hold for the Petorca data (Table A1.14). The proportion of unknowns is extremely high (58.3 percent versus only 30.2 percent for Crulai). Moreover, one must presume that in fact birth omissions are related however weakly to death omissions and consequently birth intervals following infants whose survivorship is unknown tend to be lengthened because of birth omissions resulting from temporary absences or negligence. Instead of type three intervals (unknowns) being fractionally shorter than type two (survivors), the reverse occurs for two of the four periods. Moreover, best estimates even in these cases hardly produce credible results (4 and 45 percent for 1910-1929 and 1950-1959 respectively). A zero omission rate for 1885-1909 and 1930-1949 is extremely unlikely. People's migration patterns almost guarantee some underregistration of deaths because of temporary absences.

However, before accepting this analysis as simply another shortcoming of the Petorca data, the technical application of the methods must be examined closely. In the first place, although the demographic model has hardly changed at all since initially developed by Henry, the statistical methods have become increasingly complex with successive applications. In 1967 Henry proposed an analysis of variance to determine an error rate with the best statistical fit. The technique involves successive iterations with various omission rates to determine the best estimate, i.e. the one which yields minimum statistical error. In empirical applications, however, two disconcerting quantitative anomalies arise. Both problems are

TABLE A1.14
Birth intervals according to survival status of initial infant (cumulative percentages)

Length of Subsequent Interval	Died	Survived	Unknown	Total
		Petorca, 1885-1909		
8-11	20.1	5.3	3.6	6.0
12-14	42.6	10.3	9.0	13.2
15-17	62.7	18.9	17.0	22.7
18-20	76.2	31.5	27.8	34.4
21-23	84.4	45.9	45.9	50.2
24-26	90.2	61.5	64.3	66.4
27-29	92.2	73.9	76.1	77.3
30-35	95.5	89.5	91.4	91.3
36-47	100.0	100.0	100.0	100.0
N	244	660	1262	2166
% of total	11.3	30.5	58.3	100.0
48+ (N)	13	62	124	199
Median	16.1	24.8	24.7	24.0
		Crulai, 1688-1742		
9-14	35.5	4.7	4.3	10.1
15-20	64.5	25.8	22.7	31.8
21-26	81.8	52.2	47.6	56.1
27-32	90.9	67.0	69.2	71.9
33-38	94.5	82.4	80.0	83.8
39-44	98.2	91.5	91.4	92.7
45-50	99.1	96.5	94.6	96.4
51-56	100.0	100.0	100.0	100.0
N	110	318	185	613
% of total	17.9	51.9	30.2	100.0
Median	18.0	26.5	27.7	25.5

Sources: Fertility Dataset; Gautier and Henry, La population de Crulai, p. 54.

NOTE: Petorca data includes only families with: husband born in, marriage in study area, and end of observation known (or in 1970 census). Crulai data are for Type M families and exclude intervals occurring within five years of last registered event.

related to the demographic assumptions of the model: the distribution of type three birth intervals should be greater and at shorter intervals than the distribution for type two. In practice, intervals following unknowns are sometimes longer than those after known survivors. Henry recognized this problem from the beginning and for this reason rejected a comparatively simple statistical measure, mean birth intervals, to try to reduce this risk as much as possible (and also avoid the skewness introduced by a few longer intervals). However, the use of variances involves essentially the same anomaly. An examination of relative deviations for each type of interval invariably reveals that at least half of the statistical "error" is generated where, according to the demographic model, it is least important, that is, birth intervals of thirty-nine months and longer. It is curious that the best estimate is determined statistically by elements relatively unimportant in a substantive sense.[13]

A positional measure, such as the median or a specific birth interval beyond which survival status is unrelated to subsequent fertility (say, twenty-four months), might be considered a more attractive alternative. Nevertheless, the empirical findings for both the Petorca data and the Crulai figures reported in 1958 show that for intervals of less than two years there are proportionately fewer type three cases than type two. The use of medians does not always produce logical results. The Crulai medians yield negatives--a contradiction since it indicates that deaths were overrecorded. For Petorca, possible, if not plausible, factors are generated for two other periods (1885-1909 and 1930-1949 with rates of 5.1 and 0.5 percent respectively).

Another possibility would be to compare the first interval, in which the cumulative percentage of unknowns is greater than for the survivors, and to compute the correction factor therefrom; but, this method is hardly scientific. In fact, for the Petorca data of thirty-two possible intervals for which type three cumulative percentages should be greater than type two, the expected relationship occurs in only seven instances, four of which are in one cohort (1885-1909) and are relatively tardy (intervals of two years or more). For Crulai the situation is actually worse with only one instance in eight, although a different tabulation given in 1968 is better with three out of eight in the expected direction and two for intervals of less than twenty-seven months. An extraordinary fit is found for Tourouvre au Perche, where all five of the shorter intervals show the predicted relationship and all measures (minimum variance, medians, and selection of arbitrary interval) produce almost identical results (8.2-10.7 percent underregistration).[14]

In summary, tests of infant death registration are not very successful in measuring omission rates with any precision for the Petorca Valley. They show that in general there is a marked internal consistency and that, at least, the effects of migration and negligence are not overwhelming during the period of civil registration (in contrast to that of the ecclesiastical period). After 1885 the burial data are so systematic that one may measure the influence of some very subtle social values. Subtle preferences for male offspring are revealed in the birth interval data. When a male infant died, a subsequent conception occurred twenty-four days earlier (based on medians) than following a female infant death. Conversely, when a male infant survived the first year of life, on the average a subsequent conception occurred thirty-two days later than when the survivor was a female (based on prime families for the period 1885-1969). Differential mortality rates by sex do not explain these variations (about the same proportion of females died at specific ages during the first year of life as males). People referred to the customary search for the male ("buscar el hombre"). What is surprising is that the search is quantifiable with these data which are necessarily incomplete.

With respect to specific numerical indicators of underregistration, only guesses are possible. The various tests indicate that either omissions were few, random, or disguised by birth omissions. It seems that registration of deaths must have been worse for the first civil cohort (1885-1909) with perhaps 5-35 percent of deaths not being recorded. For later cohorts omissions probably declined to between 5-20 percent, but these numbers are hunches rather than directly quantifiable assertions. The important conclusion is that the trend of mortality change for infants would not be seriously modified by any of these data corrections. If anything, the rate of mortality decline would become somewhat greater if corrections were made.

Analysis of child mortality errors is even more difficult. There are no guidelines or widely used methods other than comparisons with model life tables. Moreover, most historical demographers argue that model life tables may be inappropriate even for European historical populations. Finally, most specialists agree that levels of infant mortality correlate poorly with child mortality; consequently, it hardly seems worthwhile to wade through the quantitative paraphernalia to prove points which are more readily sustained with nonquantifiable information. The effects of omissions (through negligence or temporary absence) must be to underestimate actual rates. This fact is particularly true in the 1960s when many children began to leave the valley at early ages to attend school elsewhere. It is likely that the extremely low child mortality rates, at least for the most recent decade, are too low. It also seems likely that corrections would tend to lessen the speed of mortality decline for children as a whole (ages 1-14 years) rather than increase it.

At each step some attempt has been made to estimate the degree of disagreement between the official records and demographic realities. If absolute levels of error and bias are unknowable, the foregoing should help to appreciate probable limits.

NOTES

1. Gautier and Henry, La population de, pp. 43, 59, 98, 249-252.

2. Ramon E. Henkel, Tests of Significance (Beverly Hills, CA, 1976). D. Morrison and Ramon E. Henkel (eds.), The Significance Test Controversy (Chicago, 1970), pp. 182-198.

3. Hugo Behm, Mortalidad infantil y nivel de vida (Santiago, 1962), p. 24.

4. This table is inadvertently limited to post-1884 birth cohorts because of a mistaken limitation for this contingency table. Funds are presently unavailable to generate the table for parish data (1840-1884). Regarding Table A1.10, earlier cohorts are deliberately excluded because of the paucity of linkable infant deaths from parish burial inscriptions. Parents' names were usually omitted from parish burial registers.

5. Wrigley, "Mortality in Pre-industrial," p. 566; Gautier and Henry, La population de, p. 31.

6. See McCaa ("Chilean Social and") for a graph of these data. Odette Tacla Chamy, Panorama demográfico de Chile y su evolución en el presente siglo (Santiago, 1975), did not analyze marriage information or population structure by marital status. Juan Crocco Ferrari (Ensayos sobre la población chilena [Santiago, 1947], notes the significance of marriage for population prediction but does not go beyond a crude analysis, see pp. 68-72.

7. For a formal commentary on the visit see Libro de Bautisos VIII, f. 127; Archivo Parroquial de Petorca.

8. Adela Legareta et al., "Omissions in the Registration of Deaths in Maternity Hospitals in Santiago, Chile," Bulletin of the Pan American Health Organization, Vol. 7 (1973), pp. 35-40.

9. Wrigley, "Mortality in Pre-industrial," p. 554.

10. Wrigley, "Mortality in Pre-industrial," pp. 564-572. T. H. Hollingsworth, "The Importance of the Quality of Data in Historical Demography," Daedalus, Vol. 97 (1968), pp. 423-425. L. Henry, Manuel de démographie historique (Paris, 1967), pp. 22-25.

11. John Knodell and Hallie Kinter, "The Importance of Breastfeeding Patterns on the Biometric Analysis of Infant Mortality," Demography, Vol. 14 (1977), pp. 391-409.

12. T. E. Smith, "The Cocos-Keeling Islands: A Demographic Laboratory," Population Studies, Vol. 14 (1960), pp. 120-122.

13. Gautier and Henry, La population de, p. 54; Henry, Manuel de démographie, pp. 22-25; Charbonneau, Tourouvre-au-Perche, pp. 30-34.

14. Ibid.

APPENDIX II
Methods and Procedures

Henry elaborated the reconstitution method over a quarter of a century ago and his approach was generally applied to the Petorca data. However, there were some divergences. A particularly lamentable deviation was caused by the fact that many deaths were not linkable. Most infant deaths for the years 1860-1884 were unusable because parentage was omitted from the original documents. The problem of unfinished contemporary histories is explained in Appendix I. Finally, the reconstitution process was complicated by the frequency of natural families and the considerable variation in family names associated with illegitimacy.

All births, deaths, marriages, and wills were copied by hand from the registry books onto individual forms (4000 work hours), which were then ordered by family name and transferred to the corresponding pedigree (7000 hours). Offspring who married (as discerned from marriage or death records) were entered on two distinct family histories: once as children on that of the parents and on a second set as parents themselves. Given the never-ending advances in data input, a description of the detailed procedures used herein have only antiquarian interest. Nevertheless, it should be noted that the data were computerized at a very late stage and that consequently some information peculiar to individual acts was necessarily omitted in condensing it onto family forms. A more attractive procedure would be to transfer the data directly from the original books to computer tape, a method which was rejected at the outset as too costly. However, with the development of sophisticated linking programs and statistical packages to manipulate hierarchically structured data sets, I would no longer consider a hand operation an attractive alternative.[1] Before the data finally got to the computer they had passed through the hands of at least three research assistants and checked three times; the opportunity for error is evident.

After the pedigrees were constructed, the data were transferred to magnetic tape using the same facilities and personnel available to the Chilean Census Bureau. The computer data were then checked for illegal codes and inconsistencies by a laboriously devised FORTRAN program. Next, the histories were reordered by the female head's family name (with replicated histories for women with a second family name, or segundo apellido) to search for duplicated families resulting from orthographic variations, aliases, and name changes. This stage consisted of a four-step process: (1) the new file with the duplicated histories were sorted by women's family name(s) with a standard software package; (2) an especially written FORTRAN program selected and printed clusters with potential links; (3) I examined all clusters to determine definitive matches and coded the results as linking instructions; (4) a second FORTRAN program using the instructions developed from the hand linkages for each cluster merged duplicate families and chained together the histories of women with various consorts. The number of histories were reduced by almost 15 percent at this stage. Given the substantial incidence of illegitimacy it is essential in working with Chilean registers to reorder the histories by as many family names as possible to trap duplicates.

Most of the demographic analysis was accomplished with a combination of FORTRAN programs and procedures from the Statistical Package for the Social Sciences (SPSS).[2] Several programs were written to generate pertinent variables from the histories in a form manipulable by SPSS. (SPSS cannot manage family histories directly because of the hierarchical structure and variable length--according to the number of children of the pedigrees.) Most SPSS output was in the form of contingency tables generated with the CROSSTABS procedure.

The exceptions of more general interest were the means used to calculate fertility and mortality rates. For the fertility data set a FORTRAN program was designed to create the pertinent variables according to Henry's rules of observation, indicating the number of years at risk for each fertile age group and a paired variable specifying the number of birth events occurring at that age (15-19, . . . 45-49). The program directly created an SPSS file which included a wide range of social, demographic, and technical variables pertinent for fertility analysis (e.g. wife's age at marriage, husband's birthplace, spouse's literacy, wife's premarital conception history, manner in which family left observation, number of children born after marriage and lacking birth slips, number of children born after marriage and dying in infancy, etc.). The data set contained 1811 women and 147 variables. Sums of each pair of fertility variables (sum of years at risk and sum of birth events) provided by BREAKDOWN were then used to calculate fertility rates. This complicated approach was used to take advantage of the extraordinary tabulating flexibility of SPSS. Once the data set was constructed it was a trivial matter to produce fertility rates for a wide variety of subgroups (e.g. marital fertility age 20-24 BY age at marriage [five-year groups] BY premarital conception history BY occupation of groom BY brides' birth cohort). The data could be manipulated with extraordinary ease and confidence without special programming.

BREAKDOWN was also used for calculating infant and child mortality rates. A mortality data set was created containing a large number of age-specific mortality variables with a score indicating one of three conditions: "-1" not at risk; "0" at risk, survived; "1" at risk, died in this age group. (The variables were aged one day, one week, one month, 1-11 months, infancy [0-11 months], aged 1-4 years, 4-9, 10-14, single months through the first year, and single years through age fourteen.) Once again Henry's rules were used to determine observation status and applied through a FORTRAN program which analyzed each family history, generating the appropriate scores and other social and demographic variables. Then BREAKDOWN provided the arithmetic means of the valid scores on the mortality variables ("-1" was declared as a missing value), which was exactly the corresponding mortality rates. Once again the extraordinary flexibility of the BREAKDOWN procedure was the principal justification for not calculating the rates directly with a FORTRAN program.

Testing of all programs was accomplished by an extremely tiresome analysis of two different random samples of the family histories (initially a tiny sample of twenty-five cases, then a 10 percent set) involving the checking of actual results with answers hand computed from the same cases. A researcher with more skill, time, and efficient work habits might create specific programs to generate demographic measures directly with required classifications. In this instance, a decision was made to break all processes into tiny steps so that it would be possible to check very carefully both logical design and actual programming without the confusion and uncertainty which ensues with mammoth all-purpose programs. Shortly, flexible demographic history packages may become widely available to make many of the circumvolutions used here unnecessary.

Finally, the demographic routines developed by the Cambridge Group for the History of Population and Social Structure were not used in this instance because of the conflicts between the very particular Chilean data and the fairly rigid structure of the Cambridge package. While I had my data at Cambridge most of their demographic routines were operational, but the means of controlling for the inclusion of cases and for tabulating results for specific subsets were very difficult. The Cambridge routines are elegantly designed for the relatively impoverished inscriptions which one finds in the British registers (each entry in the parish books contains the bare minimum necessary for family reconstitution analysis with no accompanying social, economic, or other variables). They do not permit the kind of flexibility in terms of selecting and transforming cases or generating specific tables available through SPSS.

NOTES

1. Bertrano Desjardins, Pierre Beauchamp, and Jacques Legare, "Automatic Family Reconstitution: The French-Canadian Seventeenth-Century Experience," Journal of Family History, Vol. 2 (1977), pp. 56-76. Barry N. Robinson, Gary D. Anderson, Eli Cohen, and Wally F. Gazdzik have developed an SPSS related system which utilizes hierarchically structured records: Scientific Information Retrieval User's Manual (Evanston, IL, 1977).

2. Norma H. Nie, C. Hadlai Hull, Jean G. Jenkins, Karin Steinbrenner, Dale H. Bent, Statistical Package for the Social Sciences, 2nd ed. (New York, 1975).

APPENDIX III
Datasets

Marriages: All marriages known to have taken place in the study area from 1830 through 1970--6318 cases, 146 variables (including adult mortality variables).

Select Marriages: Marriages in which both spouses were born in the study area, in which the age of the bride is known, and which is the first marriage for both spouses--1941 cases, 146 variables.

Births: All children appearing in the vital registers of the study area, 1830-1970--50,432 cases, 22 variables.

Linkable Births: Same as "Births," but excluding children lacking linking information--45,138 cases, 22 variables.

Fertility: Fertility record of women with the following characteristics: married in study area between 1840-1969; first spouse death known or family linked to 1970 census; husband born in study area; woman's birthdate known--1811 cases, 147 variables.

At Risk: Mortality data for infants and children. Children born in the study area to a family for which an event subsequent to the birth of the child was found, 1885-1969--16,670 cases, 165 variables.

Deaths: All people dying in the study area, 1830-1970--18,072 cases, 17 variables.

POP70: People enumerated in the study area in the 1970 census (data obtained from census manuscripts)--4445 cases, 77 variables.

APPENDIX IV
Tables of Basic Data

TABLE A4.1
The beginnings of family life: Petorca, 1840-1969

	1840-1862	1863-1894	1895-1929	1930-1969
		Mean Age		
Female age at				
beginning fertile sexual activity*	20.9	22.6	22.2	20.2
marriage	23.0	24.7	25.3	22.7
first legitimate birth	24.5	26.1	26.7	24.0
Male age at marriage	26.8	28.1	29.0	27.4
		Variance		
Beginning sexual activity	25.38	31.15	28.32	28.58
Marriage (female)	21.82	27.93	27.91	33.44
First legitimate birth	23.88	31.45	31.13	37.45
Marriage (male)	39.15	36.98	41.48	43.70
		Number of Cases		
Beginning sexual activity	874	1115	774	1048
Marriage (female)	727	925	674	945
First legitimate birth	727	925	674	945
Marriage (male)	661	866	677	948

Dataset: Marriages.

*No control for marriage order.

NOTE: Includes first marriages for both spouses with subsequent birth in study area and known age at marriage.

TABLE A4.2
Bride's marriage age by marriage cohort and beginning type: Petorca, 1840-1969

	Age of Bride					
Beginning Type	-19	20-24	25-29	30+	Total	Age Unknown
			1840-1862			
Marriage	148	175	139	75	537	148
Pregnant at marriage	45	65	31	13	154	30
Birth(s) before marriage	72	167	130	85	454	116
Total	265	407	300	173	1145	294
			1863-1894			
Marriage	158	230	188	181	757	7
Pregnant at marriage	45	83	53	29	210	0
Birth(s) before marriage	36	140	197	172	545	4
Total	239	453	438	382	1512	11
			1895-1929			
Marriage	85	129	126	116	456	6
Pregnant at marriage	35	45	47	22	149	2
Birth(s) before marriage	21	97	183	158	459	0
Total	141	271	356	296	1064	8
			1930-1969			
Marriage	273	224	102	115	714	4
Pregnant at marriage	91	55	27	11	184	1
Birth(s) before marriage	113	177	121	185	596	5
Total	477	456	250	311	1494	10

Dataset: Marriages.

NOTE: Categories are exclusive; pregnant brides who also bore one or more children before marriage are placed in the latter group.

TABLE A4.3
Age-specific marital fertility by brides prenuptial conception history and marriage periods, 1840-1969

	No Premarital Conceptions					Some Premarital Conceptions				
	20-24	25-29	30-34	35-39	40-44	20-24	25-29	30-34	35-39	40-44
1840-1862			(1.101)					(1.131)		
Birth events	76	134	138	74	37	86	189	244	164	80
Years at risk	211.4	378.7	492.8	378.8	281.1	216.5	523.6	740.4	548.0	528.7
Corrected fertility rate	396	390	308	215	145	449	408	373	286	171
Number of women	45	88	109	88	67	46	114	160	139	120
1863-1894			(1.064)					(1.141)		
Birth events	59	106	151	113	47	42	169	196	149	76
Years at risk	137.6	345.9	490.3	407.4	322.0	107.0	399.8	552.3	449.5	354.5
Corrected fertility rate	456	338	328	295	155	448	482	405	378	245
Number of women	30	77	109	89	74	23	88	121	100	79
1895-1929			(1.000)					(1.030)		
Birth events	38	77	92	61	34	48	153	288	197	86
Years at risk	87.2	187.8	291.7	257.6	217.3	105.0	381.1	751.6	615.7	484.2
Corrected fertility rate	436	410	315	237	156	471	414	395	330	183
Number of women	19	41	63	54	50	21	80	159	136	108
1930-1969			(1.000)					(1.044)		
Birth events	110	202	147	78	22	158	276	267	187	44
Years at risk	260.4	477.1	424.0	309.7	213.8	312.1	599.1	669.9	532.0	357.2
Corrected fertility rate	422	423	347	252	103	528	481	416	367	137
Number of women	57	105	101	74	49	69	139	148	119	88

Dataset: Fertility.

NOTE: Excludes women marrying after age twenty-nine. Women are defined as not at risk during age interval of marriage to reduce distortions caused by prenuptial sexual activity. Correction factor for unregistered births is in parenthesis.

Bibliography

I. MANUSCRIPTS (All collections located in the Archivo Nacional de Chile [Santiago] except where otherwise noted):

Archivo de la Contaduria Mayor. Serie II. Catastro de 1834.

Archivo de la Intendencia de Aconcagua (San Felipe). Unorganized.

Archivo de la Provincia de los Agustinos, Escrituras, 1612-1895. Santiago.

Archivo de la Real Audiencia. Vol. 563, 2068.

Archivo del Centro de Salud de Petorca (Petorca). Unorganized.

Archivo del Registro Civil de Chincolco (Chincolco).
Libros de Nacimientos, 1895- .
Libros de Defunciones, 1895- .
Libros de Matrimonios, 1895- .
Libros de Nacidos Muertos, 1935- .

Archivo del Registro Civil de Petorca (Petorca).
Libros de Nacimientos, 1885- .
Libros de Defunciones, 1885- .
Libros de Matrimonios, 1885- .
Libros de Nacidos Muertos, 1935- .

Archivo Judicial de Petorca. All legajos consulted.

Archivo Notarial de Petorca. All volumes in Petorca and the National Archive consulted, except pedimientos de minas.

Archivo Parroquial de Petorca (Petorca).
Libros de Bautismos, 1728- .
Libros de Defunciones, 1766- .
Libros de Casamientos, 1767- .
Legajos de Informaciones Matrimoniales, 1820- .
Libro del Pósito Pío, 1870-1877.
Libros de Fábrica, 1766- .
Libros de Confirmación, 1857- .
Papeles sueltos.

British Museum (London). Add 17599, f. 48-50. [Noticias territoriales de Quillota, 1778.]

Capitanía General. Vols. 2, 27, 33, 35, 58-60, 70, 71, 92,

109, 126, 127, 146, 177, 213, 216, 223, 228, 229, 232-234, 236-238, 240, 246-248, 251-253, 255-261, 265, 267-269, 272, 273, 275-279, 573, 618, 701, 814, 909, 938, 963, 971, 983, 985, 1015, 1016, 1024, 1028, 1030, 1032.

Fondo Antiguo. Vols. 2, 34, 38, 54.

Fondo Varios. Vol. 918.

Gobernación de Petorca. Unorganized. Censo de 1865 and other volumes. Most annual reports located in Gobernacion de Petorca, Archivo de la Intendencia de Aconcagua (San Felipe); unorganized.

Ministerio de Hacienda. Vol. 8.

Instituto Nacional de Estadistica. 1970 census manuscripts for the Petorca Valley.

Ministerio del Interior. Vols. 44, 122, 225, 240, 317. Vol. 113 contains census counts for 1828-1835.

II. OFFICIAL PUBLICATIONS:

A. Censuses

Oficina central de estadística. Censo jeneral de la República de Chile levantado en abril de 1854. Santiago: Imprenta del Ferrocarril, 1858.

________. Censo jeneral de la República de Chile, levantado el 19 de abril de 1865. Santiago: Imprenta Nacional, 1866.

________. Quinto censo jeneral de la población de Chile levantado el 19 de abril de 1875. Valparaíso: Imprenta del Mercurio, 1876.

________. Sesto censo jeneral de la población de Chile levantado el 26 de noviembre de 1885. 2 vols. Valparaíso: Imprenta de la Patria, 1889-1890.

________. Sétimo censo jeneral de la población de Chile levantado el 28 de noviembre de 1895. 4 vols. Valparaíso: Imprenta Guillermo Helfmann, 1900.

Comisión central del censo. Censo de la República de Chile levantado el 28 de noviembre de 1907. Santiago: Sociedad Imprenta y Litografía Universo, 1908.

Dirección general de estadística. Censo de población de la República de Chile levantado el 14 de diciembre de 1920. Santiago: Sociedad Imprenta y Litografía Universo, 1925.

________. Resultados del X censo de la población efectuado el 27 de noviembre de 1930. 3 vols. Santiago: Imprenta Universo, 1931-1935.

Centro Latinoamericano de Demografía. Chile: XI Censo de Población (1940). Santiago: CELADE [1972].

Servicio Nacional de Estadística y Censos. XII Censo general de población y I de vivienda. 5 vols. Santiago: n.d.

Dirección de Estadística y Censos. XIII Censo de población (29 de Noviembre de 1960). Santiago: n.d.; Serie A

[1960a] and Serie B (25 vols.).
Instituto Nacional de Estadística. XIV Censo nacional de población y III de vivienda. Santiago: n.d. [1971-].

B. Vital Statistics

Oficina Central de Estadística. Anuario Estadístico de la República de Chile: Entrega Primera. Santiago: Imprenta Nacional, 1860 (also Vols. 2-17 [1848-1875], año 1911, 1920).
Dirección General de Estadística. Demografía y asistencia social año 1929. Santiago: Sociedad Imprenta y Litografía Universo, 1930 (also 1940, 1949).
Servicio Nacional de Estadística y Censos. Demografía año 1953. Santiago, 1955.
Dirección de Estadística y Censos. Demografía año 1959. Santiago, 1963 (also 1960, 1961, 1964, 1966).
Servicio Nacional de Salud. Anuario 1975 Defunciones y causas de muerte. Santiago: Ministerio de Salud, 1976. Consulted years 1970-1975.
________. Anuario 1975 Nacimientos. Santiago: Ministerio de Salud, 1976.

C. Miscellaneous Official Publications

Oficina Central de Estadística. Población calculada de la República de Chile en 1910 i Reseña del Movimiento de Población del mismo año. Santiago: Sociedad Imprenta y Litografía Universo, 1912.
________. Sinopsis Estadística de la República de Chile año 1916. Santiago: Sociedad Imprenta y Litografía Universo, 1917 (also 1925).
Dirección General de Estadística. Sinopsis Geografico-Estadística de la República de Chile 1933. Santiago: Sociedad Imprenta y Litografía Universo, 1933.

D. Other

Archivo Nacional. Censo de 1812. Santiago, 1953.
________. Impuesto Agricola. Rol de Contribuyentes (Lei de 18 de junio de 1874). 2 vols. Valparaíso: n.p., 1875.
Ministerio del Interior. Memoria Anual 1863. Santiago, 1864. The following years were consulted: 1863-1868, 1871. [Mr. Robert Oppenheimer kindly supplied these references.]
United Nations. Demographic Yearbook 1975. New York: United Nations, 1975. Consulted years: 1949-1975.

III. NEWSPAPERS

Voz de Petorca (Petorca). 1894-1953.

IV. OTHER WORKS CONSULTED:

Alvarado B., Edgardo. Estudio de los Archivos parroquiales del curato de Petorca, 1771-1810. Valparaíso: Universidad Católica de Valparaíso, 1964. Unpublished memoria para licenciatura.

Alvarez S., Julia Angélica. Estudio de los libros parroquiales de Petorca, 1811-1825. Valparaíso: Universidad Católica de Valparaíso, 1964. Unpublished memoria de prueba.

Appleman, Thomas (ed.). Thomas Robert Malthus, An Essay on the Principle of Population: Text, Sources, and Background Criticism. New York: W. W. Norton and Co., 1976.

Arriaga, Eduardo E. Mortality Decline and Its Demographic Effects in Latin America. Berkeley: Institute of International Studies, University of California Population Monograph Series Number 6, 1970.

_________. "The Nature and Effects of Latin America's Non-Western Trend in Fertility." Demography, Vol. 7 (1970), pp. 483-501.

_________. New Life Tables for Latin American Populations in the Nineteenth and Twentieth Centuries. Berkeley: Institute of International Studies, University of California Population Monograph Series Number 3, 1968.

Arriaga, Eduardo E. and Kingsley Davis. "The Pattern of Mortality Change in Latin America." Demography, Vol. 6 (1969), pp. 223-242.

Baraona, Rafael, Ximena Aranda, and Roberto Santana. Valle de Putaendo: estudio de estructura agraria. Santiago: Editorial Universitaria, 1961.

Bauer, Arnold J. Chilean Rural Society from the Spanish Conquest to 1930. Cambridge, England: Cambridge University Press, 1975.

Beaver, Steven E. Demographic Transition Theory Reinterpreted: An Application to Recent Natality Trends in Latin America. Lexington, Mass.: D. C. Heath and Company, 1975.

Behm Rosas, Hugo. Mortalidad infantil y nivel de vida. Santiago: Universidad de Chile, 1962.

Blacker, C. P. "Stages in Population Growth." Eugenics Review, Vol. 39 (1947), pp. 88-102.

Blanco, Rafael and Ranajit Chakraborty. "Consanguinity and Demography in Some Chilean Populations." Human Heredity (Basel), Vol. 25 (1975), pp. 477-487.

Borde, Jean and Mario Góngora. Evolución de la propiedad rural en el Valle del Puangue. Santiago: Editorial Universitaria, 1956.

Cabello, O. "Integralidad del registro de nacimientos y oportunidad de inscripción en Chile." Estadística, Vol. 14 (1956), pp. 302-308.

_________. "Omisión del censo de 1940 y procentaje de nacidos que no se registraron en el Registro Civil." Revista de Higiene y Medicina Preventativa, Vol. 8

(1946), pp. 3-14.
Cabello, O., Jerjes Vildosola, and Marta Latorre. Tablas de vida para Chile: 1920, 1930, 1940. Santiago: Centro Interamericano de Bioestadística, 1953.
Carlsson, Gosta. "The Decline of Fertility: Innovation or Adjustment Process." Population Studies, Vol. 20 (1966), pp. 149-174.
Carvajal, Manuel J. and David T. Geithman. "Socioeconomic Fertility Determinants in Costa Rica 1963-73." New Perspectives on the Demographic Transition. Washington, D.C.: Smithsonian Institute Occasional Monograph Series, No. 4, 1976.
Charbonneau, Hubert. Tourouvre-au-Perche aux XVIIe et XVIIIe siècles: Étude de démographie historique. Paris: Presses Universitaires de France, 1970.
Coale, Ansley J. "The Decline of Fertility in Europe from the French Revolution to World War II." In S. J. Behrman, Leslie Corsa, and Ronald Freedman (eds.), Fertility and Family Planning: A World View. Ann Arbor: University of Michigan Press, 1969.
_________. "The Demographic Transition." In United Nations, The Population Debate: Dimensions and Perspectives. Papers of the World Population Conference, Bucharest, 1974. New York, 1975, Vol. 1, pp. 347-355.
Coale, Ansley J. and Paul Demeny. Regional Model Life Tables and Stable Populations. Princeton: Princeton University Press, 1966.
Coale, Ansley J. and T. James Trussell. "Model Fertility Schedules: Variations in the Age Structure of Childbearing in Human Populations." Population Index, Vol. 40, pp. 185-258.
Collver, O. Andrew. Birth Rates in Latin America: New Estimates of Historical Fluctuations. Berkeley: Institute of International Studies, University of California, 1965.
Corporación de Fomento de la Producción. Geografía económica de Chile. Santiago: Editorial Universitaria, 1967 (rev. ed.).
Crocco Ferrari, Juan. Ensayos sobre la población chilena. Santiago: Universidad de Chile, 1947.
_________. "Movimiento de la población." In Corporación de Fomento de la Producción, Geografía Económica de Chile. Santiago: Imprenta Universitaria, 1950, Vol. 2, pp. 127-154.
Cruz-Coke, Ricardo. "A Genetic Reform of the Civil Law Computations of the Degrees of Relationship in Families." Social Biology, Vol. 24 (1978), pp. 93-99.
Daly, Herman E. "A Marxian-Malthusian View of Poverty and Development." Population Studies, Vol. 25 (1971), pp. 25-37.
Davis, Kingsley and Judith Blake. "Social Structure and Fertility, An Analytical Framework." Economic Development and Cultural Change, Vol. 4 (1956), pp. 211-235.
Desjardins, Bertrano, Pierre Beauchamp, and Jacques Legare.

"Automatic Family Reconstitution: The French-Canadian Seventeenth-Century Experience." Journal of Family History, Vol. 2 (1977), pp. 56-76.

Dupaquier, J. and M. Lachiver. "Sur les débuts de la contraception en France ou les deus malthusianismes." Anales: Economies, Societés, Civilisations, Vol. 24 (1969), pp. 1391-1406.

Easterlin, Richard A. "The Effect of Modernization on Family Reproductive Behavior." In The Population Debate: Dimensions and Perspectives. Papers of the World Population Conference, Bucharest, 1974. New York, 1975, Vol. 2, pp. 263-277.

Espinosa, Enrique. Jeografía descriptiva de la República de Chile. Santiago: Imprenta Barcelona, 1897 (4th ed.).

Eversley, D. E. C. "Review of Population Patterns in the Past." Demography, Vol. 14 (1977), pp. 539-548.

__________. "The Validity of Family and Group Statistics as Indicators of Secular Population Trends." In F. Bechhofer (ed.), Population Growth and the Brain Drain. Edinburgh, 1969, pp. 179-195.

Flandrin, Jean-Louis. Families in Former Times, Kinship, Household and Sexuality. London, 1979.

Fleury, Michel and L. Henry. Noveau manuel de dépouillement et d'exploitation de l'état civil ancién. Paris: L'Institut National D'Etudes Demographiques, 1965.

Gaskin, Katharine. "Age at First Marriage in Europe Before 1850." Journal of Family History, Vol. 3 (1978), pp. 23-36.

Gautier, Etienne and L. Henry. La population de Crulai Paroisse Normande. Paris: Presses Universitaires de France, 1958.

Gimenez, Martha E. "Population and Capitalism." Latin American Perspectives, Vol. 4 (1977), pp. 5-40.

Goldscheider, Calvin. Population, Modernization and Social Structure. Boston: Little, Brown and Company, 1971.

Grew, Raymond. "Modernization and Its Discontents." American Behaviorial Scientist, Vol. 21 (1977), pp. 289-312.

Gutiérrez, Héctor, Luís Marchant, and Odette Tacla. "Encuesta de fecundidad en Valparaíso." In Conferencia Regional Latinoamericana de Población, Actas. Mexico: El Colegio de Mexico, 1972, Vol. 1, pp. 341-346.

Henripin, Jacques. La population canadienne au début de XVIIIe siècle. Paris: Presses Universitaires de France, 1954.

Henry, Louis. Anciennes familles genevoises. Étude démographique: XVIe-XXe siècle. Paris: Presses Universitaires de France, 1956.

__________. "Interval Between Confinements in the Absence of Birth Control." Eugenics Quarterly, Vol. 8 (1961), pp. 200-211.

__________. Manuel de démographie historique. Genève-Paris: Librairie Droz, 1967.

Hicks, W. Whitney. "Economic Development and Fertility Change in Mexico, 1950-1970." Demography, Vol. 11

(1974), pp. 407-421.
Hollingsworth, T. H. "The Importance of the Quality of Data in Historical Demography." Daedalus, Vol. 97 (1968), pp. 415-432.
Hurtado Ruíz-Tagle, Carlos. Concentración de la población y desarrollo económico: el caso chileno. Santiago: Instituto de Economía de la Universidad de Chile, 1966.
Keller, Carlos. El Departamento de Arica. Santiago: Ministerio de Economía y Comercio, Censo Económico Nacional, 1946, Vol. 1.
_________. "Diccionario Económico-geográfico de la República de Chile." Unpublished manuscript.
_________. Revolución en la Agricultura. Santiago: Empresa Editora Zig-Zag, 1956.
Kirk, Dudley and Frank Oeschli. "Modernization and the Demographic Transition in Latin America and the Caribbean." Economic Development and Cultural Change, Vol. 23 (1975), pp. 391-417.
Knodell, John. "Family Limitation and the Fertility Transition: Evidence from the Age Patterns of Fertility in Europe and Asia." Population Studies, Vol. 31 (1977), pp. 219-248.
Knodell, John and Hallie Kinter. "The Impact of Breast Feeding Patterns on the Biometric Analysis of Infant Mortality." Demography, Vol. 14 (1977), pp. 391-409.
Larraín Eyzaguirre, Iván. La parroquia ante el derecho civil chileno. Santiago, 1956.
Laslett, Peter. Family Life and Illicit Love in Earlier Generations. London, 1977.
Legareta, Adela, Amparo Aldea, and Lucía Lopez. "Omissions in the Registration of Deaths in Maternity Hospitals in Santiago, Chile." Bulletin of the Pan American Health Organization, Vol. 7 (1973), pp. 35-40.
Livi-Bacci, Massimo. "Fertility and Population Growth in Spain in the Eighteenth and Nineteenth Centuries." Daedalus, Vol. 97 (1968), pp. 523-535.
Malthus, T. R. An Essay on the Principle of Population. London: J. Johnson, 1807 (4th ed.).
Mass, Bonnie. Population Target: The Political Economy of Population Control in Latin America. Toronto: Women's Press, 1976.
McCaa, Robert. "Chilean Social and Demographic History: Sources, Issues, and Methods." Latin American Research Review, Vol. 13 (1978), pp. 104-126.
Mendels, Franklin F. "Notes on the Age of Maternity, Population Growth and Family Structure in the Past." Journal of Family History, Vol. 3 (1978), pp. 236-250.
Navarro, Vicente. "What Does Chile Mean: An Analysis of Events in the Health Sector Before, During and After Allende's Administration." Millbank Memorial Fund Quarterly, Vol. 52 (1974), pp. 93-130.
Notestein, F. W. "The Economics of Population and Food Supply." In Proceedings of the Eighth International

Conference of Agricultural Economists. London: Oxford University Press, 1953, pp. 15-31.
Pinto-Cisternas, J., B. Lazo, C. Campusano, and S. Ballestros. "Some Determinants of Mating Structure in a Rural Zone of Chile, 1810-1959." Social Biology, Vol. 24 (1977), pp. 234-244.
Plank, Stephen J. and Maria Lucila Milanesi. "Fecundidad en las areas rurales de Chile." In Conferencia Regional Latinoamericana de Población, Actas. Mexico: El Colegio de Mexico, 1972, Vol. 1, pp. 408-414.
Pressat, Roland. Demographic Analysis: Methods, Results, and Applications. Chicago: Aldine-Atherton, Inc., 1972.
Quezada A., Misael and Ramiro Barrantes M. "Análisis de la endogamia en una población chilena." Revista Médica de Chile, Vol. 101 (1973), pp. 227-230.
Requena R., Mariano. "Chilean Program of Abortion Control and Fertility Planning: Present Situation and Forecast for the Next Decade." In S. J. Behrman, Leslie Corsa, and Ronald Freeman (eds.), Fertility and Family Planning: A World View. Ann Arbor: University of Michigan Press, 1969, pp. 478-489.
__________. "The Problem of Induced Abortion in Latin America." Demography, Vol. 4 (1968), pp. 785-799.
Roberts, G. W. Fertility and Mating in Four West Indian Populations. Jamaica: Institute of Social and Economic Research, University of the West Indies, 1975.
Robinson, Barry N., Gary D. Anderson, Eli Cohen, and Wally F. Gazdzik. Scientific Information Retrieval User's Manual. Evanston, Illinois: Sir, Inc., 1977.
Rodríguez Ballesteros, José. Revista de la Guerra de la Independencia. Colección de Historiadores y Documentos relativos a la Independencia Nacional. Vol. 5. Santiago, 1901. Contains census data for 1835 and 1843.
Sadie, Johannes L. "Población y mano de obra en Chile, 1930-1975." In Chile. Santiago: Centro Latinoamericano de Demografía, 1969, pp. 11-81.
Shryock, Henry S., Jacob S. Siegel, and Associates. The Methods and Materials of Demography. 2 vols. Washington, D.C.: Bureau of the Census, 1975.
Siever, Daniel. "Comment on Whitney Hicks' 'Economic Development and Fertility Change in Mexico 1950-1970.'" Demography, Vol. 13 (1976), pp. 149-152.
__________. "Recent Fertility in Mexico: Measurement and Interpretation." Population Studies, Vol. 29 (1975), pp. 341-354.
Smith, T. E. "The Cocos-Keeling Islands: A Demographic Laboratory." Population Studies, Vol. 14 (1960), pp. 94-130.
Smulevich, B. Ia. Críticas de las teorías y la política burgesas de la población. Santiago: CELADE, 1971.
Somoza, Jorge and Odette Tacla. "La mortalidad en Chile, según las tablas de vida de 1920, 1930, 1940, 1952 y

1960." In Centro Latinoamericano de Demografía, Chile. Santiago, 1969, pp. 255-286.
Stycos, J. Mayone. Human Fertility in Latin America: Sociological Perspectives. Ithaca, New York: Cornell University Press, 1968.
Sutter, J. and L. Tabah. "L'évolution des isolats de deus departments français: Loir-et-Cher et Finistere." Population, Vol. 10 (1955), pp. 645-674.
Sweezy, Alan. "Economic Development and Fertility Change." In New Perspectives on the Demographic Transition. Washington, D.C.: Smithsonian Institution Occasional Monograph Series, No. 4, 1976.
Tacla Chamy, Odette. Panorama demográfico de Chile y su evolución en el presente siglo. Santiago: INE, 1975.
Tabah, Leon and Raul Samuel. "Preliminary Findings of a Survey on Fertility and Attitudes Toward Family Formation in Santiago, Chile." In Clyde V. Kiser (ed.), Research in Family Planning. Princeton: Princeton University Press, 1962, pp. 263-304.
Tabbarah, R. B. "Toward a Theory of Demographic Development." Economic Development and Cultural Change, Vol. 19 (1971), pp. 257-276.
Teitelbaum, Michael S. "Importancia de la teoría de la transición demográfica para países en desarrollo." Demografía y Economía, Vol. 10 (1976), pp. 54-67.
Tipps, Dean C. "Modernization Theory and the Comparative Study of Societies: A Critical Perspective." Comparative Studies of Society and History, Vol. 15, pp. 199-226.
Thompson, Warren S. "Population." American Journal of Sociology, Vol. 34 (1929), pp. 959-975.
United Nations. The Population Debate: Dimensions and Perspectives. Papers of the World Population Conference, Bucharest, 1974. 2 vols. New York: United Nations, 1975.
Vidal, Jorge. "Encuesta demográfica de Cauquenes: Estudio de la fecundidad." In Chile. Santiago: CELADE, 1969, pp. 225-253.
Vivar, Teresa. Estudio de los libros parroquiales de Petorca. Valparaíso: Universidad Católica de Valparaíso, 1960. Unpublished memoria de prueba.
Villalobos R., Sergio et al. Historia de Chile. 4 vols. Santiago: Editorial Universitaria, 1974.
Walle, Etienne van de. "Les enseignements de la transition demographique Européene." Cultures et Developpement (Louvain), Vol. 7 (1975), pp. 575-585.
_________. "Marriage and Marital Fertility." Daedalus, Vol. 97 (1968), pp. 486-501.
Wrigley, E. A. "Family Limitation in Pre-industrial England." Economic History Review, Vol. 29 (1966), pp. 82-109.
_________. "Mortality in Pre-industrial England: The Example of Colyton, Devon, Over Three Centuries." Daedelus, Vol. 97 (1968), pp. 546-580.

Wrigley, E. A. "The Process of Modernization and the Industrial Revolution in England." _Journal of Interdisciplinary History_, Vol. 3 (1972), pp. 225-259.
Yrarrázaval Vera, Miguel. _Manual del Rejistro Civil para conocimiento de todos y especialmente de los oficiales del registro civil_. Valparaíso: Imprenta del Nuevo Mercurio, 1885.

Index

Dellplain Latin American Studies
Published by Westview Press

No. 8 *Studies in Spanish American Population History*, edited by David J. Robinson

No. 9 *The People of the Colca Valley: A Population Study*, Noble David Cook

No. 10 *Tierra Adentro: Settlement and Society in Colonial Durango*, Michael M. Swann

No. 11 *Andean Relfections: Letters from Carl O. Sauer While on a South American Trip Under a Grant from the Rockefeller Foundation, 1942*, edited by Robert C. West

No. 12 *Credit and Socioeconomic Change in Colonial Mexico: Loans and Mortgages in Guadalajara, 1720-1820*, Linda Greenow

No. 13 *Once Beneath the Forest: Prehistoric Terracing in the Río Bec Region of the Maya Lowlands*, B. L. Turner, II

No. 14 *Marriage and Fertility in Chile: Demographic Turning Points in the Petorca Valley, 1840-1976*, Robert McCaa

Previous Dellplain Studies
Available from University Microfilms International

No. 1 *Social Fabric and Spatial Structure in Colonial Latin America*, edited by David J. Robinson

No. 2 *New Towns for Colonial Brazil: Spatial and Social Planning of the Eighteenth Century*, Roberta Marx Delson

No. 3 *Carl Sauer's Fieldwork in Latin America*, Robert C. West

No. 4 *Studying Latin America: Essays in Honor of Preston E. James*, edited by David J. Robinson

No. 5 *First Among Equals: Great Britain and Venequela, 1810-1910*, George E. Carl

No. 6 *Amazon Economics: The Simplicity of Shipobo Indian Wealth*, Roland W. Bergman

No. 7 *The Mining Society of Potosí, 1776-1810*, Rose Marie Buechler

For Product Safety Concerns and Information please contact our EU representative GPSR@taylorandfrancis.com Taylor & Francis Verlag GmbH, Kaufingerstraße 24, 80331 München, Germany

Batch number: 10725885

Printed by Printforce, the Netherlands